STUDY GUIDE TO HUMAN ANATOMY AND PHYSIOLOGY 1

MICHAEL HARRELL, M.S.

Study Guide to Human Anatomy and Physiology 1

(First edition)

By Michael Harrell,

M.S.

Published August, 2012

ISBN: 13-9781479103515

ISBN: 10-1479103519

Dedication

To my wife for her love, dedication and support.

Table of Contents

PREFACE

Welcome everyone to your guide to Human Anatomy & Physiology!

I have been teaching college level human anatomy and physiology

for many years, as well as other courses. My other classes taught

have included: pathophysiology, biology, zoology, microbiology,

and others. In this time I have seen thousands of students. I have

learned through the years the best ways to learn the most information

in the least amount of time. There are two ways to study, smart or

hard. If you will follow my information and learn the key points of

each chapter, you will make an excellent grade in your A&P class.

In each chapter concentrate your efforts on learning the key terms.

The key terms are the ones you are most likely to see on your exams.

Learn to associate words and how to connect them.

For example, "Anatomy is the study of the structure of the human

body." Look at the key words in this sentence, anatomy and

structure. Learn how to pick out these key terms and remember

them, not the entire sentence or paragraph full of information. When given a paragraph, page or whatever; just memorize the key words and then learn how to associate them. Learn what they have in common and be able to speak from one word to the next. This will be the best way to learn your anatomy text.

I will make the assumption that anyone reading this book is taking human anatomy and physiology. You will still need your text, but more as a reference to pictures and such. This guide will give you the important information from the chapters, which will be what you are most likely to see on an exam. Sample questions will be included, which are also the most likely for you to see on an exam.

Note also that this book is not a guide for A&P lab. An anatomy lab book is little more than a book with lots of pictures in it. That is what anatomy is, memorizing parts and pieces of the body. You simply look at the picture in your book and then learn those parts on a model. You may be looking at a skull, brain, kidney, etc., it is simple memorization. This book is more to help you with the lecture.

Chapter 1

How to Learn Human Anatomy & Physiology

A Beginners Guide to Making the Grade

Here's how you're going to learn the information contained in your anatomy and physiology text. First of all, an enormous amount of information is going to come at you in a very short amount of time. Most people spend their lives avoiding science, so you probably won't be prepared. Consider how much time you would usually spend studying for a class and triple that amount. If you want to learn to apply what is ahead of you, then now is the time to start working.

Points to remember:

1. A great attitude can take you far. Any instructor prefers a C student with a good attitude over an A student with a bad attitude any day of the week. No matter how tough things get, never give your instructor a hard time. That instructor has one big power and that is the grade book. Don't forget this because I can assure you, your instructor won't.

2. Develop good study habits and don't let anything disrupt them. Human are creatures of habit, so if you get into a regular studying routine, you will probably stick with it.

3. Get rid of anything which will be a distraction to you, when you are studying. Ask yourself what is it that you always allow to draw your attention, while you are studying? Find isolation during your set time to study and don't allow anything to be close enough to you, which would cause a disruption.

4. When studying, read your notes or other study material our loud. If you are listening to the information at the same time you are reading it, you are more likely to remember it. People may think

you are crazy, but they will be the same people, who are failing the class, so don't worry about it.

5. Record yourself reading your notes with some type of audio device, so you can play this back to yourself, when you have time. Many students have long drives to school and this is time you could be listening to something helpful. Don't turn on the radio or listen to useless music, when you could be studying. Most people spend at least an hour or two in the car each day, so use this time wisely. How would you like to have an extra two hours learning every day?

6. After you feel like you understand the information, explain it to someone else. If you can thoroughly explain a topic to someone, by using complete sentences and not saying, "Ummmm", then you might just know what you are doing.

7. Make yourself a short study sheet and put it in your pocket. Whenever you have a few minutes, in between class or whatever, pull out the paper and look over it. Those minutes add up over days.

8. Draw pictures of your topics whenever possible. If you force yourself to make an illustration of structures, cells, etc., it will be easier to remember them. Try it and you will find it helps.

9. When you start to feel comfortable on the next set of test material, make up your own test. You think it's easy to make out a 100 question test? Just try it and you will see it isn't so easy. After writing your own questions, give them to a friend. When they start to tell you that they don't understand the question, you will discover it isn't as easy as you think.

10. Now this one is important people, so don't blow it! The greatest skill you can ever learn is how to listen. What is that you say? You know how to listen? Have you ever just tuned someone out? Like maybe your teacher in your last class? You can hear someone speaking, but that doesn't mean you are hearing the words. If you can't repeat exactly what the speaker just said, then you weren't listening. Most people will never master this skill and their grades will reflect it.

11. College is not something you do in your spare time. When you start college, it becomes the most important thing you have to do and life is secondary. If you can't find the time to put college first, then you may not succeed.

What you will find in this book.

The quantity of information contained in the average human anatomy and physiology text is enormous and the average person can't absorb that much information in a short period of time. What you will want to do is to learn key words and phrases for a block of information. That among other learning exercises will help you to retain information quicker and more efficiently.

In example, imagine that you just saw a movie and wanted to tell a friend about what you saw. Obviously you couldn't remember everything that happened in the movie, but you would remember things such as: key characters, important events, etc. When you have a large volume of information, what you want to do is to remember key words and know how to connect them. In other words, pick out the important words and know what they have in common. If you can connect the words by telling a story, you will probably have a reasonable grasp of the information.

If you look at the organization of any human anatomy and physiology text, they are all organized in the same manner. You will first find an overview of the book, then a section on chemistry, then the cell, etc. We will cover those topics in the same order and learn them one at a time. There is no sense in fooling around any longer, let's get started.

Chapter 2

Body Organization and Terminology

This chapter will cover basic terms you will need to use in all A&P

classes. You must learn this section if you want to have any idea of

what is happening in your class.

The first chapter of any A&P text is always an introduction to basic
material. As you read this information, concentrate on remembering
the key words. For example, when you hear the word "anatomy",
you should immediately think "structure." Any definition of
anatomy always includes the word structure, so key in on that term.
Remembering a key word will fill less space in your brain, than an
entire sentence or group of sentences.

Anatomy – the study of the structure of the human body. Learning
anatomy is nothing more than memorizing structures. For example,
you can memorize bones, muscles, nerves, etc.

Physiology – the study of the function of the human body.
Physiology is always about understanding how structures work.
When studying the heart, you can memorize the chambers, valves,
etc. and that is just the anatomy part. You can also learn how the
chambers and valves function together and that is the physiology.
So don't forget those key words and you should do well.

Levels of organization of the human body. The human body can be studied at all of these levels.

Level	Example
Chemical	DNA, carbon dioxide, oxygen, hydrogen
Organelle	mitochondria, endoplasmic reticulum
Cellular	white blood cells, muscle, osteocytes
Tissue	blood, connective, nervous
Organ	heart, liver, spleen, stomach
Organ System	cardiovascular, reproductive
Organism	human, dog

An introductory course will always ask at least one question on the order of these levels. Make sure you can list them from the smallest level (chemical) up to the highest level (organism). Occasionally an instructor will also ask for an example of each level, but that is relatively easy. Examples of each level are given above, see if you can come up with your own examples.

The next topic you will want to cover is the 11 organ systems of the body. For chapter one all you will need to know is what structures are in the system and what the basic functions are. A list of these is provided below.

The human body contains 11 organ systems and systemic anatomy is the study of those systems.

1. Cardiovascular system – heart, blood, arteries, veins. Transports materials throughout the body – like nutrients, gases, wastes, hormones, cells, etc. Also, moves heat around the body in the blood.

2. Nervous system – brain, spinal cord, nerves, sensory receptors. This is the major control system of the body. It is responsible for perceiving sensation and controlling motor functions. Other functions are: thought, emotions, memory, reasoning, etc.

3. Endocrine system – the other major controlling system of the body, which consists of many endocrine glands of the body. This system is all about hormones (chemical signals) used for communication.

4. Lymphatic system – tonsils, lymph, lymph vessels, lymph nodes, thymus gland and spleen. Functions include: fighting disease, returning fluid from tissues and absorbs fats along the GI tract.

5. Integumentary system – includes skin, hair, nails, some glands (sweat, sebaceous, ceruminous, and mammary). Protects the body, regulates temperature, keeps materials in, keeps materials out, and produces Vitamin D.

6. Digestive system – oral cavity, salivary glands, pharynx, esophagus, stomach, liver, gallbladder, pancreas, small intestine, large intestine, appendix, rectum. This system breaks down food, absorbs materials and eliminates wastes.

7. Skeletal system – bones, cartilage, ligaments, joints. The system supports the body, protects deep organs, stores materials and produces blood cells.

8. Muscular system – muscles and tendons. The system is responsible for movement of the body, maintains posture, and produces most of our body heat.

9. Respiratory system – nose, nasal cavity, pharynx, larynx, trachea, bronchi, lungs. System exchanges gases (oxygen & carbon dioxide) between the blood and the air. It is also a regulator of the body pH (hydrogen ion concentration).

10. Urinary system – kidneys, ureters, urinary bladder, urethra. This is the major waste removal system of the body. The system balances water, regulates pH and balances many materials in the body.

11. Reproductive system

Male – testes, penis, epididymis, ductus deferens, seminal vesicles, prostate gland. The system produces and transfers the reproductive cells of the male to the female and produces hormones.

Female – mammary glands, ovaries, uterus, vagina, uterine tubes. The system produces hormones, reproductive cells, provides a space for fetal development and produces milk.

In chapter 1 you will always be asked, "What is the anatomic position?" You must have a general idea of what this position is and how to use it. The way it is used is that you always assume a person is in this position unless you are told otherwise. This position is most commonly used when applying the directional terms seen below. So if you have a question which reads, "When a person is standing on their head, the eyes are considered to be what in relation to the mouth?" This is a trick question to make sure, you always assume the anatomic position. It doesn't matter if a person is upside down or not, their eyes are always superior to the mouth. The reason being, superior means closer to the top of the head, not up. Another common question asks about the palm of the hands and what direction are they facing? The palms are always facing forward which is anterior. Don't forget this position and look at a picture to remember what a person looks like, while in this position.

Anatomic position – What is this position?

Lower limbs straight, feet together, trunk of body is straight, upper limbs at sides, palms forward, fingers together, neck straight, head forward, mouth closed and eyes open. Always think of a picture from your text, showing this position.

Directional terms used in anatomy:

Superior – towards the top of the head. Superior doesn't mean up, this is very important.

Inferior – away from the top of the head. Inferior doesn't mean down.

Anterior (ventral) – towards the front of the body.

Posterior (dorsal) – towards the back of the body. On a shark's back you see a dorsal fin.

Medial – towards the midline (center) of the body. Imagine a line down the center of your body.

Lateral – away from the midline of the body.

Deep – away from the surface of the body.

Superficial – towards the surface of the body.

Proximal – towards the beginning or attached end.

Distal – away from the beginning or attached end.

You will without a doubt have several questions about directional terms on test 1. Make sure you can use these terms, because they will be used throughout the entire text.

Homeostasis

Homeostasis is defined as, "A relatively constant environment within the body." Notice the term "relatively", because this is very important. If you consider something such as your body temperature, everyone knows that 98.6 F is normal temperature for most people, but there are times when our bodies deviates from this. A small amount of deviation is acceptable as long as it is for a short period of time.

Now remember there are always two mechanisms in the body which are always working to keep us at homeostasis and they are positive and negative feedback.

Negative feedback is when the body goes against a deviation from what is normal. In other words if your body temperature starts to rise, ask yourself, "What does your body do in response?" Obviously your body will sweat when it heats up. What does sweating do to the body? Sweating cools us down to a normal temperature. What was the original stimulus? Heat. What is the body's response? Cool you down. Cooling is the opposite of heating, so this is why it is called negative feedback. Negative is when the body goes against the deviation, in other words it tries to reverse the original stimulus. Almost all feedback systems in the human body are of the negative type.

In rare cases you will see examples of positive feedback. Positive feedback is when the body allows a deviation from what is normal for a period of time. Most cases of positive feedback occur with hormones. One example is when a woman becomes pregnant a hormone called oxytocin is released in greater and greater quantities. This increase in oxytocin levels is abnormal but the body doesn't stop its release. The body will allow this release because it is needed for uterine contractions during labor. After delivery the body will stop releasing oxytocin and everything goes back to normal. Point being positive feedback is when the body goes with a deviation. You will with any doubt have questions concerning homeostasis, negative feedback and positive feedback.

Characteristics of Life

You will need to know the six characteristics of life for test one. These characteristics are used to define life itself. How do you know if something is alive? Ask yourself does it exhibit the six characteristics listed below:

1. Growth – an increase in size or number of cells.

2. Metabolism – all life has chemical reactions within it.

3. Development – all life changes through time.

4. Organization – all species have a common arrangement of structures.

5. Responsiveness – all life reacts to its environment.

6. Reproduction – nothing lives forever, it must reproduce.

     Make sure you memorize these six characteristics; you will have at least one question on these items.

Body cavities

1. Thoracic cavity – surrounded by the sternum, ribs, vertebrae, and diaphragm. Encloses the heart, lungs, thymus gland, trachea, and esophagus.

2. Pericardial cavity – surrounds the heart. It is a cavity within the thoracic.

3. Pleural cavity – one surrounds each lung. You have two pleural cavities around each lung, inside the thoracic cavity.

4. Abdominal cavity – encloses liver, gallbladder, both kidneys, stomach, pancreas, spleen, small intestine, large intestine, ureters, and other structures.

5. Pelvic cavity – encloses urinary bladder, inferior parts of ureters, part of the intestines and the ovaries and uterus of the female.

6. Abdominopelvic cavity – holds all structures found in the abdominal and pelvic cavities. This is just a combination of the abdominal and pelvic cavities.

Serous membranes

The body cavities listed above possess two membranes inside of them. One is always on the outer surface of the organ and the other will surround the first.

1. Visceral membrane – the inner membrane found on the surface of the organ inside of a body cavity.

2. Parietal membrane – the outer membrane, which surrounds the visceral membrane.

Between the two membranes serous fluid will be found. This fluid has 2 functions: reducing friction and holding the organs in place.

Planes of Sectioning

The human body and all of its contents are three dimensional objects. Any three dimensional object can be dissected in any of three ways. These planes describe how a structure was dissected and you will see these planes all throughout an anatomy text. If you understand these three planes, then you will know how a structure has been cut open.

1. Transverse/horizontal plane – separates structures into superior and inferior halves.

2. Frontal/coronal plane – separates structures into anterior and posterior halves.

3. Sagittal plane – separates structures into left and right halves.

Midsaggital – equal halves

Parasaggital – unequal halves

4 Quadrants of the abdominopelvic cavity

The abdominopelvic cavity can be separated into four chambers by using two intersecting lines at the naval. These four chambers contain organs and you need to know which organs are in those four chambers. The chambers are the upper right quadrant URQ, upper left quadrant ULQ, lower right quadrant LRQ, and lower left quadrant LLQ. You will have questions about the organs and in which quadrant they are found.

URQ – liver, gallbladder, right kidney, small intestine, large intestine, superior part of right ureter

ULQ – liver, stomach, left kidney, small intestine, large intestine, spleen, pancreas, superior part of left ureter

LRQ – large intestine, small intestine, appendix, urinary bladder

LLQ – large intestine, small intestine, urinary bladder

Body regions

The human body will be broken down into many regions and if you will learn these regions now, it will be of great help in future chapters. Many structures in the human body are named by these regions, so if you learn them now, it will be much easier to remember the names of muscles, bones, nerves, etc. Your text will contain a comprehensive list of all body regions, but test questions will usually ask about the following:

Anatomical name for regions   English interpretation

1. cephalic   head

2. cervical   neck

3. thoracic   chest

4. axillary   arm pit

5. brachial   shoulder to elbow

6. antebrachial   elbow to wrist

7. carpal   wrist

8. femoral   hip to knee

9. crural   knee to ankle

10. talus   ankle

11. digital   fingers or toes

12. acromial   shoulder

See your text for a comprehensive list.

This is all a summary of many pages in your text. Make sure you know this material.

QUESTIONS

1. List the 6 levels of organization of the human body in order from smallest to largest. Also, give an example of each level.

2. List the 11 organ systems of the human body.

3. Describe the anatomic position.

4. List the 6 cavities found in the human body.

5. What are the functions of serous membranes?

6. List the 3 planes of sectioning.

7. List the 4 quadrants of the abdominopelvic cavity and the organs found in them.

Chapter 2 – Study Questions

1. An inflammation of the body cavity surrounding a lung would be?
a. pleurisy
b. pericarditis
c. hepatitis
d. peritonitis
e. endocarditis

2. Which body system includes the spleen?
a. endocrine system
b. lymphatic system
c. reproductive system
d. integumentary system
e. digestive system

3. Which body system would include ovaries, adrenal glands and pituitary gland?
a. endocrine system
b. lymphatic system
c. reproductive system
d. integumentary system
e. digestive system

4. Which body system regulates the body through the use of hormones?
a. nervous system
b. endocrine system
c. lymphatic system
d. integumentary system
e. digestive system

5. After we eat, our blood sugar levels rise. Our body releases insulin to lower our blood sugar levels. This would be an example of what?

a. positive feedback
b. negative feedback
c. forward feedback
d. right feedback
e. none of the above

6. How do you define homeostasis?

a. the relatively constant environment outside your body.
b. the deviations seen around our body.
c. The relatively constant environment inside your body
d. all of the above
e. none of the above

7. Most feedback systems of our body are of what type?

a. negative feedback
b. positive feedback
c. loop feedback
d. higher feedback
e. lower feedback

8. Which of the following is not consistent with homeostasis?

a. When we get cold, we start to shiver
b. When we get low on water, we get thirsty
c. When our blood pressure rises, our heart rate will decrease
d. When we have blood loss, our platelets plug up tissue tears
e. When our body temperature drops, we start to sweat

9. Positive feedback is when our body tries to do what?

a. Make a deviation from homeostasis stronger and allows it.

b. Works against a deviation and makes the deviation smaller.

c. both a and b

d. neither a or b

10. If you were asked, "What are your fingers in relation to your elbow?" The correct response would be?

a. lateral

b. proximal

c. deep

d. distal

e. superior

11. If you were asked, "What is your nose in relation to your ears?" The correct response would be?

a. inferior

b. distal

c. medial

d. lateral

e. superficial

12. If you were asked, "What is your sternum is relation to your vertebral column?" The correct response is?

a. lateral

b. anterior

c. deep

d. posterior

e. lateral

13. If you were asked, "What is your brain in relation to your skull?" The answer would be _____?

a. lateral

b. anterior

c. deep

d. posterior

e. lateral

14. If you were asked, "What is your nose in relation to your mouth?" The answer would be _____?

a. superior

b. inferior

c. medial

d. superficial

e. lateral

15. If you were asked, "What is your abdominal cavity is relation to your thoracic cavity?" The answer would be_____?

a. deep

b. superior

c. inferior

d. anterior

e. posterior

16. If you were asked, "What is your knee in relation to your ankle?" The answer would be_____?

a. superior

b. inferior

c. distal

d. proximal

e. anterior

17. Your neck is also known as the _____ region?

a. epigastric region

b. axillary region

c. inguinal region

d. crural region

e. cervical region

18. The region from your shoulder to elbow is the _____ region?
a. brachial region
b. antebrachial region
c. femoral region
d. pelvic region
e. carpal region

19. The wrist region is also known as the _____ region?
a. axillary region
b. brachial region
c. digital region
d. carpal region
e. tarsal region

20. The region from your knee to your ankle is known as the _____ region?
a. crural region
b. tarsal region
c. zygomatic region
d. frontal region
e. pedal region

21. The region behind your knee is the _____ region?
a. crural region
b. popliteal region
c. zygomatic region
d. frontal region
e. pedal region

22. The bottom of your foot is the _____ region?
a. gluteal region
b. femoral region

c. lumbar region
d. thoracic region
e. plantar region

23. The area of your lower back is the _____ region?
a. cervical region
b. lumbar region
c. thoracic region
d. coccygeal region
e. sacral region

24. The area of your head is the _____ region?
a. cervical region
b. crural region
c. cephalic region
d. inguinal region
e. tarsal region

25. The back of your elbow is the _____ region?
a. olecranon region
b. inguinal region
c. cranial region
d. buccal region
e. pedal region

26. Which body cavity will you find inferior to the diaphragm?
a. pericardial cavity
b. pleural cavity
c. thoracic cavity
d. abdominal cavity
e. cranial cavity

27. Which body cavity will enclose the urinary bladder?

a. pericardial cavity
b. pleural cavity
c. thoracic cavity
d. abdominal cavity
e. pelvic cavity

28. Which of our abdominopelvic quadrants contains the gallbladder?
a. upper right
b. upper left
c. lower right
d. lower left

29. Which of our abdominopelvic quadrants contains the appendix?
a. upper right
b. upper left
c. lower right
d. lower left

30. Which of our abdominopelvic quadrants contains the spleen?
a. upper right
b. upper left
c. lower right
d. lower left

31. Which of our abdominopelvic quadrants contains the right kidney?
a. upper right
b. upper left
c. lower right
d. lower left

32. Which system is responsible for our blood cell production?

a. cardiovascular
b. muscular
c. lymphatic
d. respiratory
e. skeletal

33. The spleen, stomach and heart would be found at what level of organization?
a. chemical
b. cell
c. tissue
d. organ
e. organ system

34. Which body system is responsible for the continuation of the species?
a. cardiovascular
b. muscular
c. lymphatic
d. respiratory
e. reproductive

35. Which body system contains cartilage?
a. cardiovascular
b. muscular
c. lymphatic
d. respiratory
e. skeletal

36. Which body system is responsible for vitamin D production?
a. integumentary system
b. cardiovascular system
c. lymphatic system

d. muscular system

e. respiratory system

37. Which body system absorbs fats and returns fluid back from most tissues?

a. integumentary system

b. cardiovascular system

c. lymphatic system

d. muscular system

e. respiratory system

38. Which are our two major regulatory systems of the body?

a. respiratory and cardiovascular

b. digestive and lymphatic

c. urinary and respiratory

d. nervous and endocrine

e. integumentary and reproductive

39. Which body system removes most of our wastes?

a. digestive system

b. urinary system

c. respiratory system

d. integumentary system

e. muscular system

40. In the anatomical position, which bone of the forearm is lateral?

a. humerus

b. radius

c. ulna

d. tibia

e. fibula

41. Which plane will leave you with superior and inferior halves?

a. transverse plane

b. frontal plane

c. sagittal plane

42. Which plane will leave you with left and right halves?

a. coronal plane

b. frontal plane

c. sagittal plane

43. Which plane will leave you with anterior and posterior halves?

a. median plane

b. frontal plane

c. sagittal plane

44. Which directional term means closer to the surface?

a. anterior

b. posterior

c. lateral

d. superficial

e. deep

45. Which directional term means towards the front of the body?

a. anterior

b. posterior

c. lateral

d. superficial

e. superior

46. Which directional term means away from the top of the head?

a. inferior

b. posterior

c. lateral

d. superficial

e. superior

47. Which directional term means away from the surface?
a. anterior
b. posterior
c. lateral
d. superficial
e. deep

48. Which directional term means towards the center of the body?
a. anterior
b. posterior
c. medial
d. lateral
e. deep

49. The chest is what region of the body?
a. cervical
b. inguinal
c. femoral
d. pectoral
e. tarsal

50. The front of the elbow is what region?
a. antecubital
b. brachial
c. acromial
d. popliteal
e. sacral

CHAPTER 2 – Answers to multiple choice questions.

1. A
2. B
3. A
4. B
5. B
6. C
7. A
8. E
9. A
10. D
11. C
12. B
13. C
14. A
15. C
16. D
17. E
18. A
19. D
20. A
21. B
22. E
23. B
24. C
25. A
26. D
27. E
28. A
29. C
30. B

31. A
32. E
33. D
34. E
35. E
36. A
37. C
38. D
39. B
40. B
41. A
42. C
43. B
44. D
45. A
46. A
47. E
48. C
49. D
50. A

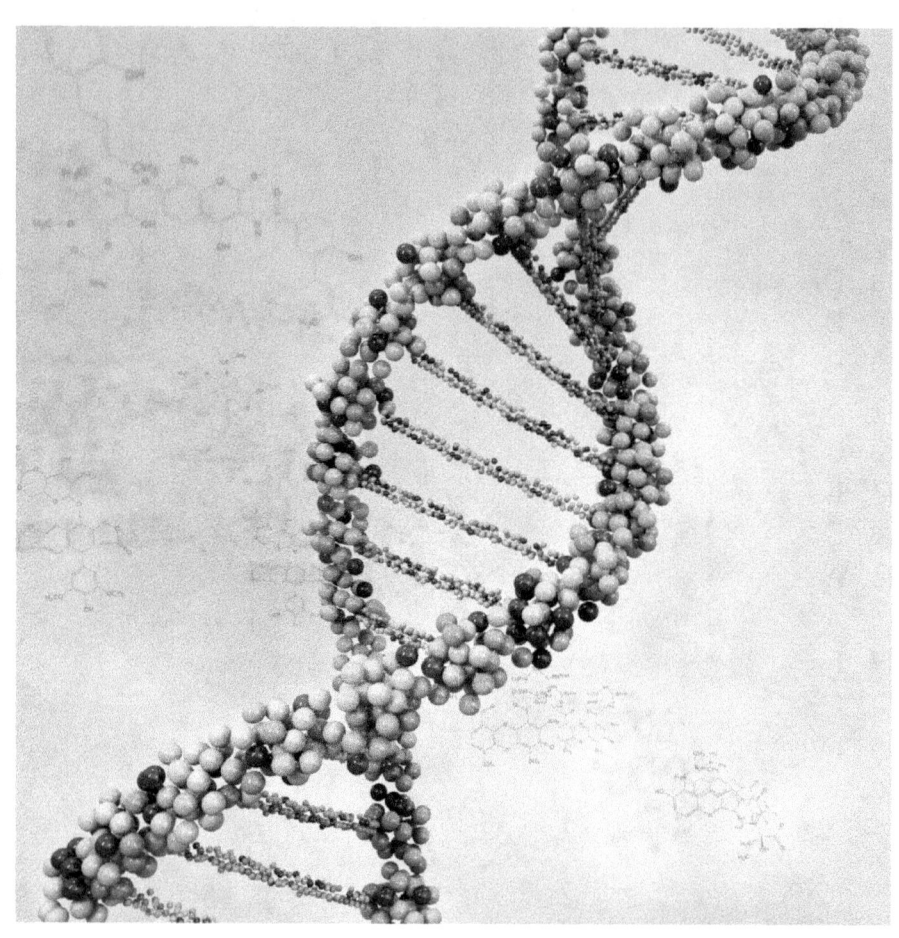

CHAPTER 3

Chemistry of the Body

The second chapter of your text will usually contain information on body chemistry. This chapter can be mastered by learning basic chemistry definitions and examples of them in the body. If you have already taken a few introductory chemistry classes, then this section should be easy for you. Some instructors will choose to skip this chapter, since it is assumed that you already know basic chemistry. You should be familiar with the following:

Again – pay attention to the key words.

1. The most common elements in the human body are: hydrogen, oxygen, carbon and nitrogen.

2. Atoms are made up of 3 subatomic particles: protons, electrons and neutrons. Make sure you know that each one has the following charges:

Protons = positive charge, found in nucleus.

Electrons = negative charge, found around the nucleus.

Neutrons = no charge, found in nucleus.

Common terms associated with the atom are:

Atomic number – the number of protons found in an atom. This is also the number of electrons found in the atom.

Mass number – the number of protons plus neutrons.

Isotopes – an element where the number of neutrons may vary.

Nucleus – the central part of an atom, which contains protons and neutrons.

Element – a substance consisting of only one type of atom. The simplest form of a substance.

Compound – a substance consisting of two or more different types of atoms.

Avogadro's number – 6.022×10^{23}

This number is used to describe the number of atoms or molecules of some substance in solution. This is how atoms are measured. We measure eggs by the dozen, water by the gallon and atoms by this number.

3. There are two types of chemical bonding: ionic and covalent.

Ionic chemical bonding occurs when electrons are swapped from one atom to another. In this type of chemical bonding, something had to lose and electron and something had to gain it. Remember, and this is a very common mistake, protons are never swapped or shared between atoms. Only the electrons are moving, during chemical bonding. This will create charged particles called ions. Two types of charged particles will exits after ionic bonding. These two particles will either be positive (cations) or negative (anions). When these ions are in water, which they always are in the human body, they will be called electrolytes. Electrolytes get this name because they conduct electricity very well.

So let's ask ourselves this, "How does sodium (Na) change into sodium ion (Na+)? Anything with a positive charge lost an electron, so anything with a negative charge had to have gained an electron. Na loses an electron to become Na+. Since it lost an electron, it now has an extra positive charge, so that is where the + comes from.

How would Cl change into Cl-? It would have to gain an electron. With the extra negative electron, this gives it the negative charge and symbol.

Covalent chemical bonding occurs when electrons are shared between atoms. After this sharing of electrons covalent bonds will be either polar or nonpolar. Remember that electrons are always shared in pairs, so either 2 or 4 are shared. This is where we get single or double covalent bonding.

Polar covalent chemical bonds occur when an unequal sharing of the electrons occurs. Water molecules are always good examples of polar covalent chemical bonding. Because of this type of bond, all water molecules are like little magnets. These little magnets are always attracting other charged particles to them.

Nonpolar covalent bonds occur when electrons are shared equally. Lipids are formed in this way and as a result don't have charges. This is why oil and water don't mix.

When chemical bonding occurs we will end up with the following materials:

Molecules – which gives us two or more atoms chemically combined. Also, remember that the combined atoms can be of the same types of materials or of different types. For example, H_2 (same atoms combined) or CO_2 (different materials combined).

Compounds – where you have two or more atoms combined, but they must be composed of at least two or more different types of atoms. For example, CO_2 and H_2O are both compounds, but H_2 isn't. H_2 is composed of only hydrogen and you must have at least two different types of atoms to be a compound.

Mass – the total of the atomic weights for any molecule or compound. If you look on the periodic table of the elements the mass for each atom is listed at the bottom. Simply add up these numbers for each atom in a molecule to get the mass.

4. Synthesis reactions – any chemical reaction in which building occurs. In other words, materials are being assembled. Anabolism is a synonym for synthesis reactions. Often water is lost by the reactants (what goes into the reaction) and a water molecule is formed. This loss of water from the reactants is called dehydration.

5. Decomposition reactions – any chemical reaction in which materials are being broken down into smaller components. Catabolism is a synonym for decomposition reactions. Often water is consumed by the reactants in decomposition reactions. This consumption of water is called hydrolysis.

In any chemical reaction always remember:

Reactants = the materials going into a chemical reaction (what was put in).

Products = what comes out of a chemical reaction (what comes out).

For example: $2H + O \rightarrow H2O$

This reads as follows: two hydrogen plus one oxygen, yields H2O (water).

Reversible reactions are chemical reactions in which you are always balancing out the materials which go into and come out of a reaction. These materials will always be trying to reach a state of equilibrium. There is one very important reversible reaction in the body and it is as follows:

$$CO2 + H2O \leftrightarrow H2CO3 \leftrightarrow H+ + HCO3-$$

This chemical reaction reads: carbon dioxide combines with water to yield carbonic acid, which dissociates into hydrogen ion and bicarbonate ion. This chemical reaction is very important because it shows the relationship between carbon dioxide and water. Always remember, whatever happens to carbon dioxide, happens to hydrogen ion. In other words, if carbon dioxide levels increase so will hydrogen ion levels. If carbon dioxide levels decrease, so will hydrogen ions. This will become very important when discussing the respiratory system and acid base balance.

6. Oxidation/Reduction Reactions

Oxidation – the loss of an electron from some material.

Reduction – the gaining of an electron by some material.

These two terms are easy to confuse. Notice that reduction is the gaining of an electron. You might ask yourself, "How is the gaining of an electron equal to reduction?" Remember that electrons have a negative charge, so if some material gains an electron, the charge is reduced. The reduction of the charge is where the term comes from.

7. Chemical Reactions

Chemical reactions in our body are affected by many variables, one such variable is temperature. As temperature increases, chemical reactions increase and just the opposite will apply also. You are likely to have a question on the topic of temperature and chemical reactions.

The concentration of reactants will also affect the speed of chemical reactions. The more reactants that are present, the faster a chemical reaction will occur. Inside of our cells we have proteins called catalysts. These proteins are what speed up chemical reactions. Chemical reaction speed is increased sometimes by a factor of one million.

8. Common inorganic materials within the human body are often discussed on the chemistry of the body. Inorganic materials are substances with don't contain carbon, but there are three exceptions to this rule. Carbon monoxide (CO), carbon dioxide (CO2), and bicarbonate ion (HCO3) are inorganic materials even though they do possess a carbon atom. Any other carbon containing compound will fit under the organic definition.

Organic materials will be any material which contains carbon except for the three compounds listed above. Common organic materials in the human body are:

a. carbohydrates – Carbs are commonly known as sugars and are a major energy source.

b. lipids – Fats are important energy storage sites and many molecules are lipids.

c. proteins – Proteins are an assembly of amino acids and perform most functions of the cells of the body. The shape of a protein is what determines its function. We must keep a relatively constant body temperature and pH to maintain proper protein shape.

d. nucleic acids – DNA and RNA are the instructions for cellular functions.

DNA is composed of four basic building blocks which only pair up in one particular way. Make sure you know cytosine always pairs with guanine, and thymine always pairs with adenine.

RNA is very similar in composition, but you will find the base thymine replaced by uracil in a RNA strand.

9. Water will be another topic in the chemistry of the body. Water is absolutely essential to life as we know it. Every chemical reaction in our body always occurs in water. Every living cell has a certain amount of water in it and around it.

Water has some certain properties, you need to be aware of. You will probably have a question concerning these properties.

First, water has a very high specific heat. What this means is that it takes a large amount of energy to change the temperature of water. Ask yourself, "How does this help us to live?" Since it takes a large amount of energy to change the temperature of water, water temperature remains relatively stable. Since it takes a large amount of energy to change the temperature of water, our body temperature remains relatively stable. We need a stable body temperature to remain healthy. If you ever wonder why there is so much discussion on temperature and pH balance in the human body, it is all about proteins. The proteins in our body determine what we can and can't do. These proteins keep their proper shape only when they are close to 98.6 F and in a pH range of 7.35 – 7.45. When we get far away from these variable, all the proteins in our bodies start to change shape. When they do we leave homeostasis and could die from it.

Think to yourself why the temperatures fluctuate so much in a desert. It can be near freezing at night and 120 degrees in the day time. The reason is, the desert has no water in it. Without water in the environment to hold the temperature stable, the temperature goes up and down quickly. If you compare this to an area where there is lots of water, you will see temperature fluctuations of about 25 to 30 degrees. Since we have so much water in our bodies, we remain at a relatively constant temperature. That is very important to maintaining homeostasis.

Water also provides protection to our body. In many joints we have fluid providing lubrication to reduce friction. Around our brain and spinal cord we have a fluid barrier to act as a shock absorber.

Remember that water is where all chemical reactions take place in our bodies.

Along with water, you will have discussions on solutes and solvents. In the body water is always the solvent in which other things are mixed into. Solvents are anything dissolved into the solvent.

10. Osmolality – the number of particles in a solution. You will see this term used in reference to many movement processes such as diffusion, osmosis and sensory receptors. When discussing how much of a material is found in a solution, osmolality is the term you will use. Osmolality will be expressed in a unit of measure called moles. The more moles you have, the more of a material is found in a solution. The normal osmolality of most human tissues is 300 milliosmoles.

11. pH scale – a way to measure the concentration of hydrogen ions in a substance. Don't forget that normal pH of the human body is between the range of 7.35 – 7.45. If the body pH drops below 7.35 a

condition called acidosis will develop. Acidosis is when the body contains too many hydrogen ions. If the body goes above 7.45 a condition called alkalosis develops. Alkalosis is when the body contains too few hydrogen ions.

Acid – a substance which releases hydrogen ions, also called a proton donor.

Base – a substance which accepts hydrogen ions, also called a proton acceptor.

A buffer is a substance equal in concentrations of acid and base. With its pH of 7, it is considered neutral and will neutralize and acid or a base.

You will probably have a question concerning the pH scale also. The pH scale runs between zero and fourteen. Any number less than 7 will be an acid and any number greater than 7 will be a base. Only a 7 on the pH scale is considered to be neutral. So, the number 6.99999 is what? Acid. The number 7.0000001 is what? Base.

12. Salts – a salt is any positive ion chemically bonded with an anion. So put any positive and negatively charged particles together and you have a salt. Don't forget there is one exception to this rule, water. Water is not a salt. Usually when we think of a salt, we think of NaCl. That is only one example of a salt. NaCl is a salt because it is a sodium ion (which is positive) and a chloride ion (which is negative) chemically combined.

13. You will most certainly have a few questions about the building blocks of DNA and RNA. Always remember that DNA is composed of four nucleotides called: cytosine, guanine, adenine and thymine. And they only pair up as follows: cytosine will only pair with guanine, and adenine will only pair with thymine. Don't forget how they pair up, that will be important.

RNA is very similar in its structure. It still has four nucleotides, but one of them is different. It still has cytosine and guanine paired together, but adenine pairs with uracil. Don't forget these base pairs and how they match up.

QUESTIONS

1. What is the difference between ionic and covalent chemical bonding?

2. What are the 4 most common elements in the human body?

3. What is the difference between a synthesis and decomposition reaction?

4. What are the 4 categories of organic compounds found in the human body?

5. What does RNA contain that DNA doesn't?

CHAPTER 3 QUESTIONS

1. Which of the following is not one of the four most common elements in our body?
a. nitrogen
b. oxygen
c. hydrogen
d. carbon
e. calcium

2. Which element do we need to transport oxygen in our body?
a. nitrogen
b. copper
c. iron
d. iodine
e. potassium

3. All organic molecules have what element in them?
a. nitrogen
b. oxygen
c. hydrogen
d. carbon
e. calcium

4. Which of the following elements do we need to synthesize thyroid hormone?
a. nitrogen
b. oxygen
c. iron
d. iodine
e. potassium

5. Which is not a subatomic particle found in an atom?

a. proton

b. electron

c. neutron

d. Dalton

e. none of the above

6. Which subatomic particle has a negative charge?

a. proton

b. electron

c. neutron

d. Dalton

7. The difference in elements is based on the number of _____ in them?

a. proton

b. electron

c. neutron

d. Dalton

8. How does a sodium atom become a sodium ion?

a. it gains a proton

b. it loses a proton

c. it gains an electron

d. it loses an electon

e. it gains a neutron

9. What type of chemical bonding involves the swapping of electrons?

a. ionic

b. covalent

c. polar covalent

d. nonpolar covalent

e. hydrogen bonding

10. What type of chemical bonding involves the sharing of electrons?

a. ionic

b. covalent

c. hydrogen

d. anabolism

e. catabolism

11. Water molecules are formed by what type of chemical bonding?

a. ionic

b. covalent

c. polar covalent

d. nonpolar covalent

e. hydrogen bonding

12. Sodium and chloride will form a salt by what form of chemical bonding?

a. ionic

b. covalent

c. hydrogen

d. anabolism

e. catabolism

13. The materials that go into a chemical reaction are called the what?

a. catabolites

b. metabolites

c. reactants

d. products

e. electrons

14. The materials which are produced from a chemical reaction are called the what?
a. catabolites
b. metabolites
c. reactants
d. products
e. electrons

15. A chemical reaction that can shift from left to right, or right to left is called a ___ reaction?
a. standard reaction
b. opposite reaction
c. reversible reaction
d. decomposition reaction
e. synthesis reaction

16. A chemical reaction in which smaller parts are assembled together is a _____ reaction?
a. standard reaction
b. opposite reaction
c. reversible reaction
d. decomposition reaction
e. synthesis reaction

17. A chemical reaction is which a larger material is broken down into smaller materials is a _____ reaction?
a. standard reaction
b. opposite reaction
c. reversible reaction
d. decomposition reaction
e. synthesis reaction

18. Anabolism is the same as a
a. standard reaction
b. opposite reaction
c. reversible reaction
d. decomposition reaction
e. synthesis reaction

19. The mixing medium for all chemical reactions inside the human body is?
a. sodium
b. oxygen
c. water
d. carbon
e. hydrogen

20. What do you call any ion in water?
a. metabolite
b. acid
c. base
d. electrolyte
e. salt

21. The pH scale runs between what 2 numbers?
a. 0-10
b. 0-100
c. 2-8
d. 0-14
e. 10-100

22. On the pH scale any number less than 7 will be considered a what?
a. acid

b. base

c. salt

d. electrolyte

e. metabolite

23. On the pH scale any number greater than 7 will be considered a what?

a. acid

b. base

c. salt

d. electrolyte

e. metabolite

24. An acid may also be called a what?

a. proton acceptor

b. proton donor

c. electron donor

d. electron acceptor

e. none of the above

25. Which is not an example of an organic molecule?

a. carbohydrate

b. lipid

c. protein

d. nucleic acid

e. water

26. On the pH scale a number 7 is considered?

a. an acid

b. a base

c. neutral

d. organic

e. inorganic

27. What best defines a lipid?

a. a polar molecule

b. a complex carbohydrate

c. a simple sugar

d. a nonpolar molecule

e. an important component of DNA

28. Which element is not found in carbohydrates?

a. oxygen

b. iron

c. carbon

d. hydrogen

29. Which is not a function of lipids in the body?

a. energy storage

b. padding around organs

c. heat insulator

d. structure of important molecules

e. component in DNA

30. The building blocks of all proteins are?

a. carbohydrates

b. lipids

c. amino acids

d. nucleic acids

e. simple sugars

31. The number of protons plus neutrons is?

a. atomic number

b. mass number

c. total number

d. neutral number

e. largest number

32. The subatomic particles not found in the nucleus are?
a. protons
b. neutrons
c. electrons
d. all of the above
e. none of the above

33. When electrons are shared equally, this is what type of chemical bonding?
a. ionic
b. nonpolar covalent
c. polar covalent
d. hydrogen bonding
e. total bonding

34. Which of the following materials will release Hydrogen ions?
a. acid
b. buffer
c. base
d. protein
e. lipid

35. What is the normal pH range for the human body?
a. 0-14
b. 7.35-7.45
c. 0-10
d. 6.5-7.5
e. 6-8

36. If a person breathes too rapidly, they won't have enough hydrogen ions in their blood. What condition will result from low hydrogen ion levels?
a. acidosis
b. alkalosis
c. metabolism
d. sucrose
e. hyperventilation

37. What are the 4 nitrogenous bases found in DNA?
a. cytosine, guanine, uracil, adenine
b. guanine, thymine, cytosine, adenine
c. uracil, thymine, guanine, adenine
d. cytosine, guanine, adenine, uracil
e. thymine, cytosine, uracil, adenine

38. What are the 4 nitrogenous bases found in RNA?
a. cytosine, guanine, uracil, thymine
b. guanine, thymine, cytosine, adenine
c. uracil, thymine, guanine, adenine
d. cytosine, guanine, adenine, uracil
e. thymine, cytosine, uracil, adenine

39. Which nitrogenous base is found in RNA but not DNA?
a. cytosine
b. guanine
c. adenine
d. thymine
e. uracil

40. Which nitrogenous base is found in DNA but not RNA?
a. cytosine
b. guanine

c. adenine

d. thymine

e. uracil

41. The energy molecule for cells is

a. adenosine triphosphate

b. adenosine biphosphate

c. adenosine monophosphate

d. lipids

e. ribonucleic acid

42. Which ion is needed for muscle contraction, blood clotting and bone strength?

a. nitrogen

b. oxygen

c. hydrogen

d. carbon

e. calcium

43. What part of the atom contains the protons and neutrons?

a. isotope

b. nucleus

c. electron cloud

d. triglyceride

e. peptide

44. Two or more forms of an element with different numbers of neutrons?

a. isotope

b. nucleus

c. electron cloud

d. triglyceride

e. peptide

CHAPTER 3 – Answers to multiple choice questions.

1. E
2. C
3. D
4. D
5. D
6. B
7. A
8. D
9. A
10. B
11. C
12. A
13. C
14. D
15. C
16. E
17. D
18. E
19. C
20. D
21. D
22. A
23. B
24. B
25. E
26. C
27. D
28. B
29. E
30. C

31. B
32. C
33. B
34. A
35. B
36. B
37. B
38. D
39. E
40. D
41. A
42. E
43. B
44. A

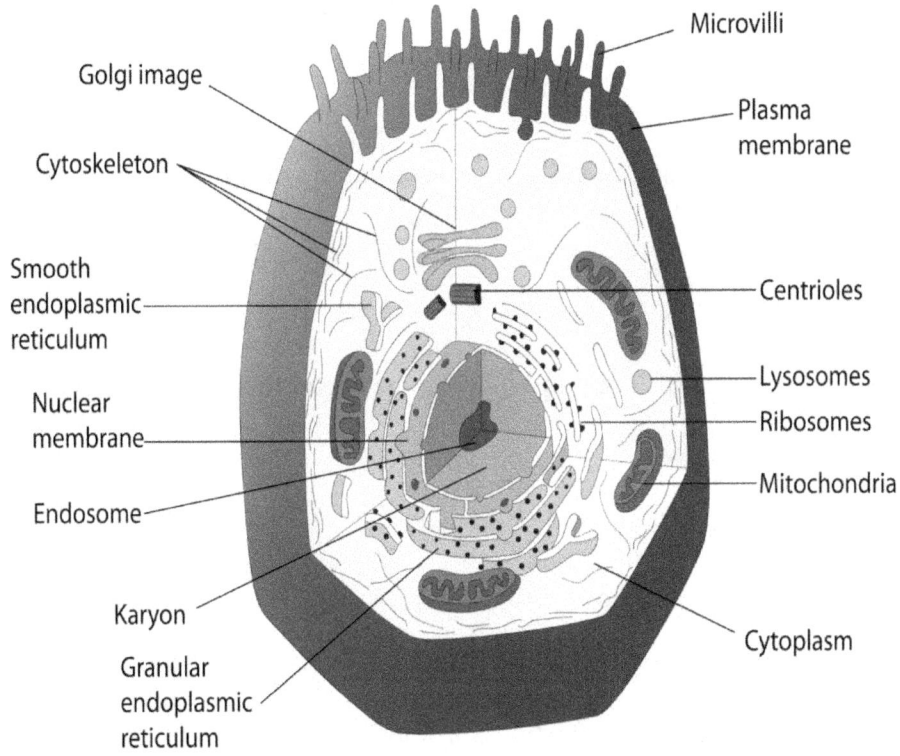

Golgi image

Cytoskeleton

Smooth endoplasmic reticulum

Nuclear membrane

Endosome

Karyon

Granular endoplasmic reticulum

Microvilli

Plasma membrane

Centrioles

Lysosomes

Ribosomes

Mitochondria

Cytoplasm

CHAPTER 4

Cell Anatomy and Physiology

The next section of your text will cover the cell. The cell chapter will discuss the structures of the cell, what the functions of these structures are, how materials move in and out of the cell and cellular division.

The cell will be described as the fundamental unit of all living things and is nothing more than many chemicals working together. This is the lowest level of organization in which all of the characteristics of life can be observed.

Cytology is the study of cells. Diseases can be traced to some type of cellular change. Your text will illustrate what is normal for a cell, so when you study diseased states, you will have a basis in which to compare them to.

The cell consists of 3 main parts: plasma membrane, nucleus, and cytoplasm.

1. Plasma membrane – outer boundary of cell, interface between cell and environment.

What can pass through plasma membrane? Water (through channels only!), nutrients, oxygen, ammonia, carbon dioxide, ions, metabolic products. Where water must pass through channels, lipids may diffuse freely through the plasma membrane. If ever asked which material (water or lipid soluble materials) can pass through the cell membrane, you answer, "lipids". Remember that the cell membrane is about half lipids, so anything else that is a lipid will pass through it, because lipids and lipids will mix.

The outside of the cell is called the extracellular environment and the inside is called the intracellular environment. This cell membrane will have a charge which results from ion concentration differences. Ions (charged particles) give the cell membrane a charge. The cell will pump more of the positive ions (Na, Ca) to the outside of the cell and have more negatively charged particles (PO4, proteins) on the inside. This gives the cell a positive charge on the outside and a negative charge on the inside. Don't forget this information, it will be very important when you discuss action potentials (electric charges).

When you look at any picture of the cell membrane you will always see two things in those pictures, lipids and proteins. The proteins are the structures penetrating the cell membrane. The lipids are all of the tiny structures in between them. The lipids are there as a barrier, while the proteins are there for many reasons.

Phospholipid bilayer – What is it made of? ½ protein, ½ lipids, small amount of carbohydrates.

The plasma membrane will be described as being neither hard and rigid or fluid. This is the fluid mosaic model of the cell membrane. This means that even though the cell membrane does make a barrier around the cell, it is always changing.

Be sure and know the basic types of ion channels, which are found in cell membranes. These ion channels are:

A. nongated (leak) channels – these channels are always open and whatever material they are particular to may pass freely whenever they need.

B. ligand gated ion channels – a ligand is chemical signal, which is the same as a drug, hormone, neurotransmitter, etc. These types of channels will open or close in response to a chemical signal.

C. voltage gated ion channel – action potentials (electric signals) will open or close these gates.

Know these ion channels, they will be very important in future discussions, especially when it comes to muscle cells and neurons. These electrically excitable cells will be using these ion channels to generate action potentials (electric signals).

Movement process through the cell

A. Diffusion – this is simply the movement of materials from an area of high concentration to low. In other words, atoms move from where there are more of them to where there are less of them. Think of the smell of cookies diffusing from the kitchen to the living room or the smell or an orange as someone beside you peels it. Inside the body oxygen, carbon dioxide and many other materials move by diffusion. This process moves more materials than any other process in the body.

B. Osmosis – think of osmosis as the diffusion of water. Water moves from high to low concentrations, just like many other materials. Also, remember that water always moves towards solute concentrations. Where ever solutes are in highest concentration, the water will move towards it. The cell doesn't pump water but it does move solutes and the water follows it.

C. Active transport – active transport will always involve the use of ATP to move something through the cell membrane. Think of ATP as fuel for proteins in the cell membrane. As this ATP is consumed, materials are moved in and out of the cell. Many proteins in a cell membrane are there to move materials from one side of the cell to the other. The most common example of active transport in the body is the sodium/potassium exchange pump. Every time this protein uses up an ATP molecule it will pump out three sodium ions and pump in two potassium. This pump is what is largely responsible for setting up the resting membrane potential (the charge found on a cell membrane).

D. Endocytosis – to bring something in to the cell.

2 types of endocytosis – phagocytosis (cell eating), pinocytosis (cell drinking).

E. Exocytosis – when the cell moves something out of it, through the use of vesicles (a little ball of material inside the cell).

F. Filtration – filtration is the movement of some material across a membrane with tiny holes in it. You will see this in places like the kidneys. When you think of filtration, think of the filter on a coffee pot. You use the filter to hold back large particles, but it lets the water and tiny particles pass through it.

Proteins in the cell membrane, which move materials, are often placed into three categories.

Uniporters – proteins which move one material at a time.

Symporters (cotransporters) and Antiporters (countertransporters) those that move two materials at a time. The difference between the two is: symporters move two materials in the same direction. The materials may be moved into the cell or out. Antiporters move materials in opposite directions. One goes in while the other goes out. These two transporters will only work if a concentration gradient (a difference in the concentration of a material) exists. So, an active transporter will set up this concentration gradient and then the transporters will work second. This is why symport and antiport are called secondary active transporters. They will only work if an active transporter is already working.

Enzymes – proteins which lower activation energy and speed up chemical reactions. It's important for enzymes to lower activation energy, otherwise, it would take more energy to start a reaction, than we would get out of it.

2. Nucleus - 2 major functions-A) houses the genetic information, B) controls the tasks of the cell. These 2 tasks are carried out by DNA.

Nuclear membrane - double membrane with nuclear pores. Allow copies of genetic material to pass.

Nucleoli - portions of chromosomes that make ribosomes.

The nucleus is involved with the production of proteins, since this is where the set of instructions for making them is found. You will always see two processes in the making of proteins. Transcription will take place in the nucleus and translation will take place in the cytoplasm at a ribosome.

Nuclear pores – holes which materials allow materials to pass in and out of the nucleus.

Chromatin – the form of our DNA when the cell is not dividing. This is the thin strand form and how our DNA is found for most of the cell's life.

Nucleoplasm – this is the fluid and materials inside the nucleus. Like the cytoplasm is the fluid and materials in the cell, the nucleoplasm is the fluid and materials in the nucleus.

3. Cytoplasm – all of the material inside of the cell but outside of the nucleus.

Consists of 3 things – cytosol (fluid portion), cytoskeleton (framework of the cell), and organelles (tiny organ like structures).

Other structures

Vesicles – fluid filled sacs – 3 functions – digest subcellular material, transport material out of the cell, and carry on enzymatic activities.

Also protects the integrity of the plasma membrane. Vesicles can fuse with the cell membrane and ejects materials out of the cell.

3 specialized vesicles

A. Lysosomes – digest material by phagocytosis, which means cell eating. Digested materials may come from outside or inside of the cell.

B. Peroxisomes – detoxify $H_2O_2 \rightarrow H_2O + O$. Breaks down hydrogen peroxide into water and oxygen.

C. Proteasomes – digests proteins into amino acids.

Cytoskeleton – Gives the cell shape and can move things. The cytoskeleton is like the skeletal and muscular systems of the cell.

ORGANELLES

Organelle means tiny organ and think of each one of these structures as a tiny little factory, which provides one or more functions within the cell. You will undoubtedly have many questions concerning these structures.

1. Mitochondria – these are all about ATP production think of them as the power plants of the cell. The mitochondria also house a small amount of genetic information, just like the nucleus.

2. Ribosomes – the sites of protein synthesis. Think of these as the factories where proteins are made. Ribosomes are found in two ways. They may be attached to a rough endoplasmic reticulum or found free in the cytoplasm. No matter where they are found, they will always be producing proteins. Those on the rough endoplasmic reticulum are making proteins to go out of the cell. The free ribosomes are making proteins to stay inside of the cell.

3. Endoplasmic Reticulum – these are networks of enclosed sacs.

2 types A. rough ER – these have ribosomes attached to the surface (this is what makes them look rough), these structures produce proteins for use outside of the cell.

B. smooth ER – these don't have ribosomes on the surface, produces lipids, detoxifies material, store calcium.

4. Golgi apparatus or Golgi body – modifying, packaging, distributing site of the cell. After lipids and proteins are produced by other organelles, they are sent here for further modification.

5. There are many types of vesicles which may be found inside of a cell. A vesicle is just a little ball of material inside of the cell. Vesicles come in many forms and you can't tell them apart visually. Each vesicle contains a different material, with a different function.

Vesicle types are:

-Lysosomes – these vesicles contain digestive enzymes, so they act as the digestive system of the cell.

-Proteasomes – these vesicles contain enzymes needed to digest proteins.

-Peroxisomes – detoxify harmful materials inside of the cell.

6. Centrioles – structures associated with spindle fiber formation during mitosis. These gear shaped structures are surrounded by a region called the centrosome. The centrosome is where spindle fibers will appear during mitosis. These organelles are important during cellular division.

Other structures – extensions of plasma membrane and microtubules

7. cilia – move materials over the surface of cells like mucus.

8. flagella – propels the cell. Think of these as like an outboard motor on the back of the cell. These are the largest and fewest in number of the external structures.

9. microvilli – these structures increase surface area where you need absorption and secretion. These are the smallest and greatest in number of the external structures.

THE CELL CYCLE – This consists of the stages a cell goes through in its life span.

3 events – Interphase, Mitosis, Cytokinesis

1. INTERPHASE – growth and DNA replication is occurring. Interphase is not part of mitosis, don't forget this.

3 phases

A. G1 phase – growing and producing organelles.

B. S phase – synthesis, DNA replicated.

C. G2 phase – grows and prepares for mitosis.

2. MITOSIS – nuclear division

4 phases

A. Prophase – chromatin condenses into chromosomes, and each chromosome has 2 arms called chromatids, which are connected at the centromere.

What else will you see occurring in prophase?

-Nucleolus disappears

-nuclear membrane disassembles

-mitotic apparatus appears – consists of spindle fibers, attached at the centromere in a region called the kinetochores and astral fibers radiate to each pole.

B. Metaphase – chromosomes align across the center of the cell (equator of cell). When you see the chromosomes in a nice line, this phase has started.

C. Anaphase – chromatids separate at centromere and these structures are called daughter chromosomes. When you can see the chromosomes being pulled in half, this phase has started. Spindle fibers will pull daughter chromosomes toward poles.

D. Telophase – daughter chromosomes reach poles and the cell can be seen separating in half into 2 new daughter cells. Other things seen are:

-Cytokinesis begins (division of the cytoplasm)

-Chromosomes unwind into chromatin

-Nucleolus reappears

-Nuclear envelope reforms

-Mitotic apparatus disassembles

3. Cytokinesis – splitting of the cytoplasm. This is division of everything but the nucleus.

Begins in late anaphase or early telophase

Cleavage furrow – plasma membrane constricts

Protein synthesis

Your text will generally have a small amount of information on how proteins are produced. You will learn much more information on this topic in microbiology.

Proteins are made in three simple steps:

A. Transcription – To transcribe something means to copy it. When a cell wants to make a protein the first thing it needs is a recipe to follow. This recipe is obtained from the nucleus, when a small part of the DNA is copied. This copy is called mRNA, the m stands for messenger. Think of this as your recipe.

B. Translation – To translate the mRNA, the cell must take it to the ribosome out in the cytoplasm. Remember the ribosomes are the sites of protein synthesis. Think of the ribosome as the kitchen for making the protein.

C. Protein synthesis – The building of the protein will occur in the cytoplasm at the ribosome. A molecule called tRNA (transfer RNA) will bring in amino acids one at a time. The tRNA knows where to place an amino acid, according to the information on the mRNA.

Highlights to remember:

-Steps are: transcription, translation, protein synthesis

-Transcription occurs in the nucleus.

-Translation occurs in the cytoplasm.

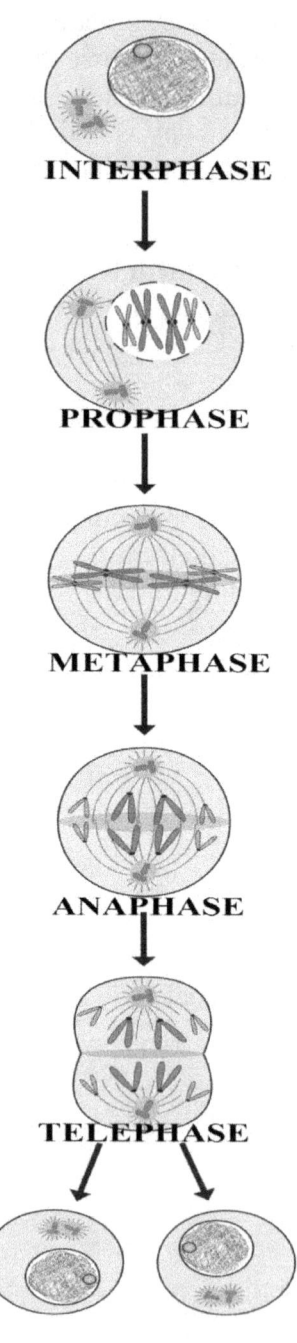

INTERPHASE

PROPHASE

METAPHASE

ANAPHASE

TELEPHASE

QUESTIONS

1. List the organelles of the cell and the major functions of each.

2. List and describe the stages of the cell cycle.

CHAPTER 4 – QUESTIONS

1. The functional unit of all living organisms is?
a. cell
b. tissue
c. organ
d. DNA
e. RNA

2. The 3 main parts to any cell are?
a. DNA, RNA, ATP
b. cell membrane, nucleus, DNA
c. cytoplasm, DNA, RNA
d. cell membrane, nucleus, cytoplasm
e. none of the above

3. The cell membrane is also called the?
a. plasma membrane
b. phospholipid membrane
c. fluid mosaic model
d. cell barrier
e. all of the above

4. The cell membrane is made primarily of 2 materials. These 2 are?
a. lipids and carbohydrates
b. lipids and proteins
c. proteins and DNA
d. proteins and carbohydrates
e. DNA and carbohydrates

5. The phospholipids found in the cell membrane have?
a. a polar head region
b. 3 tails on the nonpolar region
c. 3 polar head regions
d. polar regions facing the inside of the cell
e. non polar regions facing the intracellular and extracellular regions

6. Tiny work stations inside the cell are called?
a. cytosomes
b. endosomes
c. proteins
d. organelles
e. none of the above

7. Which organelle of the cell produces most of the ATP?
a. nucleus
b. vesicles
c. lysosomes
d. Golgi body
e. mitochondria

8. Which organelle of the cell is responsible for calcium storage, lipid production and detoxification?
a. nucleus
b. vesicles
c. smooth endoplasmic reticulum
d. Golgi body
e. mitochondria

9. Which organelle is responsible for protein synthesis?
a. nucleus
b. rough endoplasmic reticulum
c. smooth endoplasmic reticulum

d. Golgi body

e. mitochondria

10. Which organelle is responsible for breaking down proteins?

a. nucleus

b. rough endoplasmic reticulum

c. smooth endoplasmic reticulum

d. Golgi body

e. proteasomes

11. Which organelle is responsible for housing most of the genetic materials?

a. nucleus

b. rough endoplasmic reticulum

c. smooth endoplasmic reticulum

d. Golgi body

e. proteasomes

12. Which organelle is responsible for modifying, packaging and distributing materials out of the cell?

a. nucleus

b. rough endoplasmic reticulum

c. smooth endoplasmic reticulum

d. Golgi body

e. proteasomes

13. Which organelle acts as the digestive system of the cell?

a. lysosomes

b. rough endoplasmic reticulum

c. smooth endoplasmic reticulum

d. Golgi body

e. proteasomes

14. When the cell is at rest the intracellular charge will be?

a. positive

b. negative

c. neutral

d. none of the above

15. When the cell is at rest the extracellular charge will be?

a. positive

b. negative

c. neutral

d. none of the above

16. What is it called when the cell membrane swaps the charges on its surface?

a. transduction

b. mitosis

c. diffusion

d. depolarization

e. repolarization

17. When the cell returns to the original resting charge this is called?

a. transduction

b. mitosis

c. diffusion

d. depolarization

e. repolarization

18. The charges on the cell membrane come from what materials?

a. lipids

b. carbohydrates

c. ions

d. DNA

e. RNA

19. What is the most abundant ion found in the human body?
a. potassium
b. sodium
c. calcium
d. phosphate
e. magnesium

20. What is the most abundant cation (positive) ion found in the extracellular environment?
a. potassium
b. sodium
c. calcium
d. phosphate
e. magnesium

21. What is the most abundant cation found in the intracellular environment?
a. potassium
b. sodium
c. calcium
d. phosphate
e. magnesium

22. What protein in the cell membrane is primarily responsible for setting up the resting membrane potential?
a. calcium pumps
b. hydrogen pumps
c. sodium – potassium exchange pumps
d. potassium pumps
e. chloride pumps

23. Why does the rough endoplasmic reticulum look rough?

a. It has DNA on its surface.
b. It has lipids on its surface.
c. It has ribosomes on its surface.
d. It has lysosomes on its surface.
e. It has peroxisomes on its surface.

24. Vesicles leaving the cell will be sent out from what organelle?
a. nucleus
b. rough endoplasmic reticulum
c. smooth endoplasmic reticulum
d. Golgi body
e. mitochondria

25. Cell eating of solid particles is called?
a. endocytosis
b. pinocytosis
c. phagocytosis
d. exocytosis
e. none of the above

26. Cell drinking is called?
a. endocytosis
b. pinocytosis
c. phagocytosis
d. exocytosis
e. none of the above

27. When the cell brings materials into the cell, this is called?
a. endocytosis
b. pinocytosis
c. phagocytosis
d. exocytosis
e. none of the above

28. To take something out of the cell is called?

a. endocytosis
b. pinocytosis
c. phagocytosis
d. exocytosis
e. none of the above

29. Tiny containers of materials found inside of the cell are called?

a. ribosomes
b. vesicles
c. lysosomes
d. organelles
e. plasmasomes

30. The folds seen inside mitochondria are called?

a. cisternae
b. peptides
c. matrix
d. cristae
e. Golgi bodies

31. Besides the nucleus where else can DNA be found?

a. nucleus
b. rough endoplasmic reticulum
c. smooth endoplasmic reticulum
d. Golgi body
e. mitochondria

32. Most cells will have one, centrally located what?

a. nucleus
b. rough endoplasmic reticulum

c. smooth endoplasmic reticulum
d. Golgi body
e. mitochondria

33. When our cells are not dividing, our genetic material is found in what form?
a. protein
b. chromatin
c. cytoplasm
d. nucleoplasm
e. cytoskeleton

34. The small structure inside the nucleus, which houses RNA is?
a. nucleolus
b. chromatin
c. cytoplasm
d. nucleoplasm
e. cytoskeleton

35. The fluid environment inside the nucleus is called?
a. DNA
b. chromatin
c. cytoplasm
d. nucleoplasm
e. cytoskeleton

36. What process can be used to move materials through the cell membrane?
a. diffusion
b. active transport
c. endocytosis
d. exocytosis
e. all of the above

37. Why does the cell prefer to use diffusion to move materials?
a. diffusion doesn't require energy use
b. diffusion moves materials in to the cell
c. diffusion moves materials out of the cell
d. diffusion can move water
e. none of the above

38. Which transport mechanism requires the expenditure of ATP?
a. diffusion
b. active transport
c. endocytosis
d. exocytosis
e. all of the above

39. The movement of materials from an area of high to low concentration is?
a. diffusion
b. active transport
c. endocytosis
d. exocytosis
e. all of the above

40. The movement of water from areas of high to low concentration is?
a. diffusion
b. active transport
c. endocytosis
d. exocytosis
e. osmosis

41. The structures inside of the cell which give it shape and form are?

a. cytoplasm
b. cytoskeleton
c. sarcolemma
d. mitochondria
e. endoplasmic reticulum

42. What transport mechanism allows oxygen and carbon dioxide to move in and out of the lungs?
a. diffusion
b. active transport
c. endocytosis
d. exocytosis
e. osmosis

43. What transport mechanism moves more materials than any of the others?
a. diffusion
b. active transport
c. endocytosis
d. exocytosis
e. osmosis

44. What organelles are cylinder shaped and involved with moving materials during mitosis?
a. nucleus
b. rough endoplasmic reticulum
c. smooth endoplasmic reticulum
d. Golgi body
e. centrioles

45. The fluid environment inside the cell is called?
a. nucleus
b. rough endoplasmic reticulum

c. cytoplasm

d. centrosome

e. mitochondria

46. A region of the cytoplasm where centrioles can be found is the?

a. nucleus

b. rough endoplasmic reticulum

c. smooth endoplasmic reticulum

d. centrosome

e. mitochondria

47. A structure found on the outside of a cell and used to move the cell is?

a. cilia

b. microvilli

c. flagella

d. all of the above

e. none of the above

48. Structures found on the outside of the cell and used to move materials over the surface of the cell?

a. cilia

b. microvilli

c. flagella

d. all of the above

e. none of the above

49. Structures on the outside of the cell, used to increase surface area for absorption or secretion?

a. cilia

b. microvilli

c. flagella

d. all of the above

e. none of the above

50. Which of the following materials can pass through the cell membrane at any time?

a. proteins

b. lipids

c. carbohydrates

d. ions

e. nucleic acids

51. Which of the following materials cannot pass through the cell membrane by diffusion?

a. water

b. lipids

c. estrogen

d. testosterone

e. cholesterol

52. The smell of perfume moving through a room is an example of?

a. diffusion

b. active transport

c. endocytosis

d. exocytosis

e. all of the above

53. An increase in temperature will do what to diffusion rate?

a. increase it

b. decrease it

c. has no effect

54. An increase in solute concentrations will do what to diffusion rate?

a. increase it
b. decrease it
c. has no effect

55. A decrease in molecule size will do what to diffusion rate?

a. increase it
b. decrease it
c. has no effect

56. Two containers are separated by a selectively permeable membrane. Solution 1 contains 4 grams of solutes and solution 2 contains 9 grams of solutes. In which direction will water move?

a. from 1 to 2
b. from 2 to 1
c. net movement will be the same
d. none of the above

57. A hypotonic solution contains _____ solutes than a hypertonic solution?

a. more
b. less
c. same

58. Most tissues of the human body have what concentration of solutes?

a. 500 milliosmoles
b. 200 milliosmoles
c. 1000 milliosmoles
d. 300 milliosmoles
e. 20 milliosmoles

59. A transport mechanism which only works after active transport and moves two materials in the same direction is?
a. diffusion
b. osmosis
c. cotransport (symport)
d. countertransport (antiport)
e. facilitated diffusion

60. A transport mechanism which only works after active transport and moves two materials in the opposite direction is?
a. diffusion
b. osmosis
c. cotransport (symport)
d. countertransport (antiport)
e. facilitated diffusion

61. The cytoplasm is
a. material inside of cell and outside of nucleus.
b. material inside of nucleus
c. material outside of cell

62. The process by which the cell destroys and recycles old organelles is?
a. mitosis
b. autosome
c. autophagia
d. anaphase
e. telophase

63. Which of the following is not a stage of mitosis?
a. interphase
b. prophase
c. metaphase

d. anaphase

e. telophase

64. In which stage of cell division does chromatin condense into chromosomes?

a. interphase

b. prophase

c. metaphase

d. anaphase

e. telophase

65. In which stage of cell division does cytokinesis begin?

a. interphase

b. prophase

c. metaphase

d. anaphase

e. telophase

66. In which stage of cell division do the chromosomes form a line at the equator of the cell?

a. interphase

b. prophase

c. metaphase

d. anaphase

e. telophase

67. In which stage of cell division do the chromosomes split and migrate apart?

a. interphase

b. prophase

c. metaphase

d. anaphase

e. telophase

68. After mitosis cells will enter which of the following stages?
a. interphase
b. prophase
c. metaphase
d. anaphase
e. telophase

69. After mitosis the two daughter cells will have?
a. a full set of DNA
b. half set of DNA
c. two sets of DNA

CHAPTER 4 – Answers to multiple choice questions.

1. A
2. D
3. E
4. B
5. A
6. D
7. E
8. C
9. B
10. E
11. A
12. D
13. A
14. B
15. A
16. D
17. E
18. C
19. B
20. B
21. A
22. C
23. C
24. D
25. C
26. B
27. A
28. D
29. B
30. D

31. E
32. A
33. B
34. A
35. D
36. E
37. A
38. B
39. A
40. E
41. B
42. A
43. A
44. E
45. C
46. D
47. C
48. A
49. B
50. B
51. A
52. A
53. A
54. A
55. A
56. A
57. B
58. D
59. C
60. D
61. A
62. C
63. A

64. B
65. D
66. C
67. D
68. A
69. A

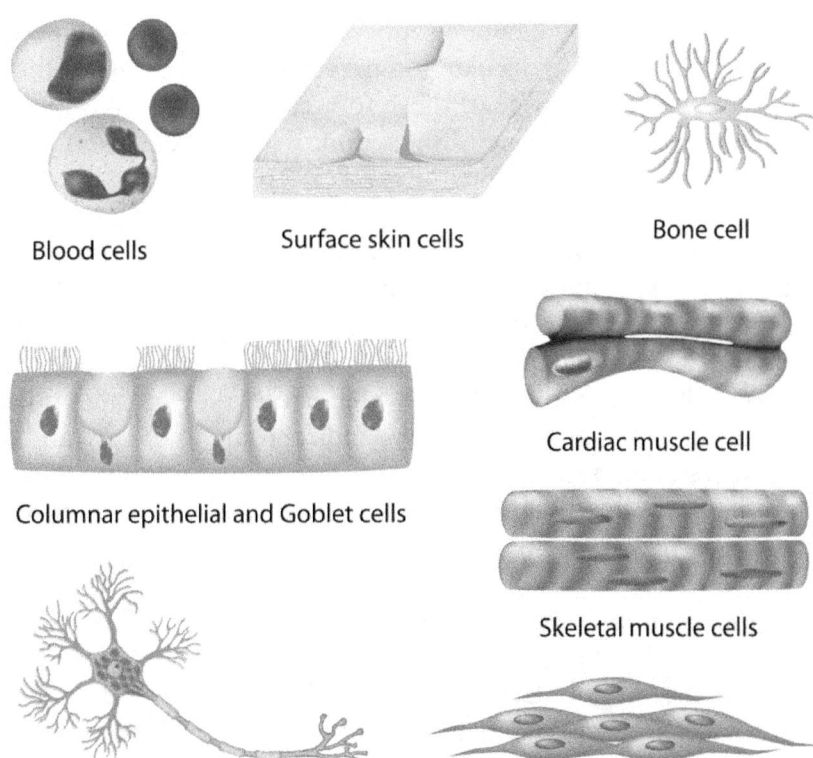

Blood cells

Surface skin cells

Bone cell

Columnar epithelial and Goblet cells

Cardiac muscle cell

Skeletal muscle cells

Neuron

Smooth muscle cells

CHAPTER 5

Tissues

Tissue – a collection of cells, plus their surrounding material (matrix).

There are many tissue types in the human body and we want to discuss the primary tissues.

The tissues in our body can be grouped into 4 different categories: epithelial, connective, muscular and nervous. Every tissue of the body can be placed into one of these four categories. Make sure you can place any tissue into one of those four tissue types.

1. EPITHELIAL TISSUE

Epithelial tissue will be found in many places of the body. Primarily you will find it covering and lining most surfaces of the body. Skin will come to mind first and that is a great example of epithelial tissue. Remember this tissue is found in many places. If you look at the four body systems which open to the outside of the body (respiratory, digestive, urinary, and reproductive) they all have passageways opening to the outside of the body. All of these passageways are lined with epithelial tissues. Also, most glands of the body are made of epithelial tissue.

Even though this tissue is creating a barrier in many places, don't think that they don't allow for the passage of materials. In some places, like the skin, the cells allow very little to pass through them. In many other places they do allow for passage. Thick layers will always prevent the passage of materials, where thin layers will allow for passage.

Epithelial tissue always has certain characteristics. Make sure you are familiar with the characteristics of each of the tissues. In epithelial tissues you will see the following:
- Very little space between the cells. Epithelial cells are tightly packed, so they can make good barriers. Some of these binding connections are desmosomes, hemidesmosomes, gap junctions and tight junctions. Other tissues are not as tightly packed as epithelial tissues are.
- Most epithelial tissues will have a structure called the basement membrane. This is a thin layer which will bind it to another tissue and guides it during cellular repair. Not all epithelial tissues have it,

but it is a characteristic of most. A basement membrane won't be found with any other tissue type.
- Blood vessels don't penetrate epithelial tissues. Why is this? Many epithelial tissues are superficial and on the surface of something. Since they are superficial, you don't want blood vessels penetrating them. If blood vessels did, it would be easy to lose blood and get infections into them.
- Epithelial tissues have many proteins binding them together. With all of these binding structures, it holds them together tightly, making a good barrier.
-Because these cells are covering and protecting structures, the cells are always being lost on their surface. Because of this, the cells are almost always in mitosis.

A few terms will describe most epithelial tissues and you need to know what the terms mean. There are three terms which describe epithelial cell layers and three which describe cell shapes.
The three terms describing cell layers are:
Simple – 1 layer
Stratified – 2 or more layers
Pseudostratified – 1 layer. The term means falsely stratified, because it looks like two layers. This type will often have cilia on the surface and mucous is often what the cilia are moving. They will often have goblet cells with them. Goblet cells do one thing, make mucous.

The three terms describing cell shapes are:
Squamous – means flat
Cuboidal – cube shape
Columnar – tall and thin, like a column in front of a house
In the description of most epithelial tissues you will find one word from the first group and one word from the second group. Examples would include:
Simple squamous epithelial tissue = one layer of flat cells
Simple columnar = one layer of column shaped cells
Stratified squamous = many layers of flat cells
Make sure you understand the meaning of these six terms. You will without a doubt, have questions concerning the meaning of each.

Another type of epithelial tissue, which the above terms don't describe are transitional epithelial tissue. This special type of epithelial tissue is capable of changing its number of cell layers and cell shape. That is why it's called transitional. If something is going through a transition, it is changing. This special tissue is found in the urinary system and allows for expansion. Your urinary bladder has to be able to expand, if it is to fill with urine.

Where you find epithelial tissues making glands, you will find them in two types.
Endocrine glands – glands found within the body producing hormones. These glands will be discussed in detail when you get to the endocrine system. These glands release their products into the spaces surrounding the cells and enter the blood.

Exocrine glands – glands with a duct leading to the surface of something. Many of these glands are found in the skin. Examples would be sweat glands, sebaceous (oil) glands, mammary glands and ceruminous (ear) glands.
    Exocrine glands come in three forms:
-Merocrine – glands which use exocytosis (vesicles) to secrete materials. Ex-sweat glands
-Apocrine – glands which pinch off a piece of their cell with the materials in them. Ex-mammary glands
-Holocrine – glands were the entire cell falls away into the duct. Ex-sebaceous glands
Make sure you know how the materials are released and an example of each.

2. CONNECTIVE TISSUE
    Connective tissue is the most varied tissue in function and number of locations. There are more tissues within this category than any of the others by far. If you are ever asked to place a tissue into a category and you don't know where it goes, then put it in this one. Connective tissues can often be found connecting other tissues

together, thus the name. For example, tendons connect bones to muscles, ligaments connect bone to bone, blood connects most tissues of the body, etc. Many other functions can be performed by this tissue.

Inside the connective tissues you will find an abundance of extracellular matrix. This means that there is much more space between the cells. This is the opposite of epithelial tissue, which has little extracellular space.

The cell names of connective tissues have some terms within them, you need to be familiar with. In connective tissue cell names you will find the suffixes: blasts, clasts and cytes. Any cell name with blast in it will be a building cell, any with clast in its name will be a breaking down cell and any cyte cell will maintain a tissue. For example, in bones you will find three big cell types: osteoblasts, osteoclasts and osteocytes. Osteoblasts build bone, osteoclasts break down bone and osteocytes maintain bone (meaning the build small amounts). Don't forget those suffixes, they can serve you well in determining cell physiology.

Along with the cells of connective tissues, you will also find several common fibers.
- Collagen is the most common connective tissue fiber and the most abundant protein in the body. Collagen gives strength to tissues. Think of them as steel cables. A steel cable will bend but it won't stretch, this is where the strength comes from.

-Elastin (elastic) fibers are a common fiber which is very flexible. Think of elastin fibers as rubber bands. These fibers will stretch and give flexibility to things such as your arteries.

-Reticular fibers are a type of fine collagen, found mostly in the lymphatic system.

Connective tissues found in the body include the following:

- Adipose tissue – this is what we commonly call fat tissue. Adipocytes are the fat cells you find in adipose tissue. We have adipose tissue to store energy, insulate the body (hold in heat) and make a cushion around deeper structures. In the first few years of our lives we have a special type of adipose tissue called brown adipose tissue. It is specialized to produce heat in the body.

- Bone tissue – Bone is the hardest, densest tissue in the body. Because it is so hard it is often found protecting deeper structures. Bone comes in two types: compact and cancellous.
Compact bone is a type of bone where the tissue is very compact, with no spaces within it. When you see a histology slide of this bone, it is the one that looks like tree stumps. You will find compact surrounding all bones.
   Bone is composed mostly of two materials: collagen (1/3) and hydroxyapatite (2/3). The collagen gives our bones flexibility and the hydroxyapatite makes it hard.
Cancellous bone is also called spongy bone, because it looks a bit like a sponge. Think about all the spaces found within a sponge, which is what this bone looks like.

- Reticular tissue is a tissue full of reticular fibers. If you want to find this tissue, look to the lymphatic system and bone marrow.

- Loose connective tissue - also called areolar tissue. This tissue gets its name because the fibers have lots of space in between them. Look at any picture of loose connective tissue and you will see all the space between the fibers.

-Dense connective tissue – This tissue gets its name because the fibers are tightly packed together. This tissue is the opposite of the loose tissue. Dense tissue can be found as regular or irregular. Regular dense connective tissue is where most of the fibers are oriented in the same direction, like in a tendon or ligament. Irregular dense connective tissue is where most of the fibers are oriented in many directions.

-Elastic tissue – where the tissue is filled with elastic fibers. This tissue will stretch very well. Arteries have large amounts of elastic tissue in them. Our vocal cords have dense regular elastic tissue.
- Blood – The only tissue in the body that flows like a fluid, because it has so much water in its matrix. Blood connects almost all tissues of the body. Blood is composed of plasma (the watery part of the blood) and the formed elements (the cells of the blood). Blood cells will consist of red blood cells, white blood cells and platelets.

- Hemopoietic tissue – This tissue is what we commonly call bone marrow. This is where all of the blood cells are made. There are two types of bone marrow in the body. When we are young we have red bone marrow, but as we pass maturity, we have more yellow bone marrow. They are the same tissue but yellow marrow has more adipose tissue in it and red has less adipose tissue.

- Cartilage – This is a strong tissue composed of cells called chondrocytes. Cartilage doesn't contain blood vessels or nerves. Since this tissue is often found in pressure points, it would be useless to put blood vessels and nerves in them. Three types of cartilage are found in the body.
    Hyaline cartilage – This is the second strongest tissue in the body, just after bone. In between bones where they meet and the embryo skeleton are common sites for this tissue.
    Elastic cartilage – A type of tissue which contains large amounts of elastic fibers. The ears and nose have large amounts of this tissue. That is why those body parts are so flexible.
    Fibrocartilage – Cartilage found in joints under high compression. The disks in between the bodies of our vertebrae are good examples of this tissue. This tissue forms cushions in some joints, acting as shock absorbers. If you ever felt something pop in your knee or jaw, that was fibrocartilage.

3. MUSCLE

Muscle comes in three forms in the body.

Skeletal – This is the most abundant of the 3 muscle types and is always attached to bone. Skeletal muscle makes about 40% of our total body weight. It has more than one nucleus (peripherally located), had bold stripes on it (striations), is under voluntary control and has a round shape like a pipe. This muscle is what we move our body parts with.

Cardiac – This muscle is only found in the heart. In the heart it's generating pressure to move our blood. These cells have one nucleus, are centrally located and are round in shape. This muscle is involuntary, meaning you can't control it with your conscious thought.

Smooth muscle – This muscle is found in more locations than any other muscle type. Because it is found in so many places, its functions are varied. Much of it is in our digestive system, that is what moves materials through our GI tract. This muscle has a spindle shape to the cells. It has one nucleus per cell and is also involuntary.

4. NERVOUS TISSUE

The nervous system contains many cells, but the most important ones are the neurons. These are what you may call brain cells, but they are found in many places other than the brain. A neuron has 3 main parts to it. These parts are the cell body (soma), dendrite (where neurons receive signals) and the axon (the output part of the neuron).

In addition to the neurons you will find a group of cells called glial or neuroglial cells. These are any cell in the nervous system that isn't a neuron. They are varied and have many functions. When we get to the nervous system, we will go over them.

Neurons are also classified in different ways. One classification is based on the structure of the cell. Some neurons have many dendrites (multipolar cells), some have one dendrite (bipolar cells) and some have no dendrites (unipolar cells). The number of dendrites is all that varies in this structural classification. The bipolar and unipolar are easily confused. Bipolar get their name because they have two poles, one input (1 dendrite) and one output (1 axon). Unipolar only have an axon, thus unipolar.

Epithelial tissues of the body form membranes in many areas and you need to know them.

1. Serous membranes – These are the same membranes discussed earlier in chapter 2. The membranes which surround organs and are found in enclosed body cavities. The pericardial, pleural and peritoneal cavities have these visceral (inner) and parietal (outer) membranes. The membranes and fluid reduce friction and hold the organs in place.

2. Mucous membranes – These are the membranes lining the body systems, which have openings to the outside of the body. The linings of the respiratory, digestive, urinary and reproductive systems all have these membranes.

3. Synovial membranes – These membranes will be found in some of the joints of the body. The membrane will release a fluid containing hyaluronic acid. This acid makes the cartilage in the joints very slippery and this will reduce friction.

Inflammation
    When a tissue is damaged for any reason, it will become inflamed. Inflammation is caused by materials moving from the cardiovascular system into the tissue. When tissues are damaged, chemicals of inflammation are released. These chemicals work to make blood vessels dilate (bringing more blood into a tissue) and make the vessels more permeable (allowing more to move out of the blood). You want more blood in a damaged tissue for the following reasons:

1. Bringing in more red blood cells, delivers more oxygen to cells, which will be needed for repair.
2. Bringing in more white blood cells, will allow for more dead cells and foreign invaders to be destroyed.
3. Bringing in more platelets will help to stop blood loss.
4. Bringing in more plasma will bring in many materials.

The signs of inflammation are: redness, heat, pain, swelling and disturbance of function.

QUESTIONS

1. What are the 4 major tissue types found in the human body?

2. What 3 terms describe the number of cell layers found in epithelial tissue?

3. What 3 terms describe the shapes of epithelial cells?

4. What are the 3 major muscle types and where are they found?

5. What are the 3 major regions of a neuron?

6. What 3 types of fibers are found in connective tissue?

7. What is the name of the hard material found in bone?

Chapter 5 – Questions

1. A tissue is defined as _____?
a. a group of chemical working together
b. a group of cells plus the extracellular matrix
c. a group of atoms working together
d. a group of organs working together
e. a group of organ systems working together

2. The study of tissues is _____?
a. cytology
b. histology
c. endocrinology
d. pathology
e. pathophysiology

3. Which of the following is not one of the four major tissue types?
a. epithelial
b. connective
c. muscular
d. nervous
e. stem

4. What are the embryonic cells, which later develop into the adult tissues?
a. epithelial
b. connective
c. muscular
d. nervous
e. stem

5. Which tissue type is found covering surfaces and forming many glands?
a. epithelial
b. connective
c. muscular
d. nervous
e. stem

6. The outer layer of your skin is which tissue type?
a. epithelial
b. connective
c. muscular
d. nervous
e. stem

7. Which term describes an epithelial cell with a flat shape?
a. squamous
b. cuboidal
c. columnar
d. transitional
e. stratified

8. Which term describes an epithelial cell with a cube shape?
a. squamous
b. cuboidal
c. columnar
d. transitional
e. stratified

9. Which term describes an epithelial cell with a tall, thin shape?
a. squamous
b. cuboidal
c. columnar

d. transitional

e. stratified

10. Which term describes an epithelial tissue with one layer of cells?

a. simple

b. stratified

c. squamous

d. transitional

e. keratinized

11. Which term describes an epithelial tissue with multiple layers of cells?

a. simple

b. stratified

c. squamous

d. transitional

e. keratinized

12. Which term describes an epithelial tissue with one cell layer, but looks like two?

a. pseudostratified

b. stratified

c. squamous

d. transitional

e. keratinized

13. Which of the following would describe the outer layer of your skin?

a. simple squamous

b. stratified cuboidal

c. transitional

d. stratified squamous with keratin

e. moist stratified squamous

14. What type of epithelial tissue are you most likely to find in the kidneys?
a. simple squamous
b. simple cuboidal
c. simple columnar
d. stratified squamous
e. stratified cuboidal

15. Most stratified epithelial tissues have what shape?
a. squamous
b. cuboidal
c. columnar
d. simple
e. stratified

16. What special type of epithelial tissue is found in the urinary bladder?
a. simple squamous
b. stratified cuboidal
c. transitional
d. stratified squamous with keratin
e. moist stratified squamous

17. Gas exchange in the lungs, happens across what type of epithelial tissue?
a. simple squamous
b. stratified cuboidal
c. transitional
d. stratified squamous with keratin
e. moist stratified squamous

18. What is the function of a goblet cell?

a. moisture production

b. sodium production

c. mucous production

d. keratin production

e. oil production

19. Epithelial tissues never have _____?

a. flat cells

b. multiple cell layers

c. mucous coverings

d. blood vessels

e. tall, thin cells

20. Epithelial tissue in the outer layer of our skin contains a tough protein called?

a. proteoglycans

b. keratin

c. mucous

d. lipids

e. collagen

21. What does an exocrine gland have that an endocrine gland doesn't?

a. a duct

b. multiple cell layers

c. collagen fibers

d. elastic fibers

e. water

22. What type of exocrine gland secretes materials by exocytosis?

a. apocrine

b. holocrine

c. merocrine

23. What type of exocrine gland secretes materials by pinching of a piece of the cell?
a. apocrine
b. holocrine
c. merocrine

24. What type of exocrine gland secretes materials by releasing the entire cell into a duct?
a. apocrine
b. holocrine
c. merocrine

25. What structure will you find in epithelial tissue, but none of the other tissue types?
a. collagen fibers
b. reticular fibers
c. proteoglycans
d. blood
e. basement membrane

26. Cilia, microvilli and flagella will only be found on what tissue type?
a. epithelial
b. connective
c. muscular
d. nervous
e. stem

27. Which surface feature is used to increase surface area for absorption or secretion?

a. cilia

b. microvilli

c. flagella

d. organelles

e. nucleus

28. Which surface feature is used to move materials over the surface of the cell?

a. cilia

b. microvilli

c. flagella

d. organelles

e. nucleus

29. Which surface feature is used to propel the cell?

a. cilia

b. microvilli

c. flagella

d. organelles

e. nucleus

30. What tissue type is found in every organ of the body?

a. epithelial

b. connective

c. muscular

d. nervous

e. stem

31. What tissue type contains more tissues than any other?

a. epithelial

b. connective

c. muscular

d. nervous

e. stem

32. Which of the following is not a connective tissue?
a. blood
b. bone
c. adipose
d. cartilage
e. muscle

33. What connective tissue cell suffix means "building type of cell?"
a. blast
b. clast
c. cyte

34. What connective tissue cell suffix means "breaking down type of cell?"
a. blast
b. clast
c. cyte

35. What connective tissue cell suffix means "maintaining type of cell?"
a. blast
b. clast
c. cyte

36. What the most common connective tissue fiber?
a. collagen
b. elastic
c. reticular

37. Which connective tissue has large spaces in between cells and fibers?
a. dense
b. loose
c. regular
d. muscular
e. nervous

38. Tightly packed tissue with little space between the cells and fibers?
a. dense
b. loose
c. regular
d. muscular
e. nervous

39. What connective tissue has so much fluid between the cells, it flows like a fluid?
a. loose connective tissue
b. fibrocartilage
c. blood
d. cancellous bone
e. muscle

40. Which of the following is not a connective tissue cell?
a. white blood cell
b. adipocyte
c. chondrocyte
d. fibroblast
e. muscle cell

41. Which connective tissue molecule is good for trapping water?
a. collagen

b. elastic

c. reticular

d. proteoglycans

e. areolar

42. Which of the following is not a function of adipose tissue?

a. acting as a cushion for deeper structures

b. insulating the body

c. storing energy

d. producing cartilage

e. releasing energy

43. Where in the body will we find elastic tissue?

a. bone

b. blood

c. arteries

d. muscle

e. neurons

44. Which type of connective tissue contains osteons?

a. bone

b. blood

c. arteries

d. muscle

e. neurons

45. What is the function of an osteoblast?

a. to build bone

b. to bread down bone

c. to release calcium

d. to maintain bone

e. none of the above

46. What is the function of a fibroblast?

a. to build bone

b. to build muscle

c. to build fibers

d. to build macrophages

e. to build fats

47. Which is an example of dense, regular, collagenous connective tissue?

a. bone

b. ligaments

c. blood

d. muscle

e. adipose

48. Osteocytes live inside of bone in spaces called?

a. matrix

b. lacunae

c. canaliculi

d. central canals

e. osteons

49. Cancellous bone contains many interconnecting structures called?

a. collagen fibers

b. proteoglycans

c. osteons

d. compact bone

e. trabeculae

50. What type of bone development forms the flat bones of the skull?

a. endochondral

b. intramembranous

51. In what type of tissue does the production of our blood cells occur?
a. hemopoietic tissue
b. blood
c. cartilage
d. dense regular connective tissue
e. all of the above

52. Cartilage tissue is built by what cells?
a. hemopoietic cells
b. chondroblasts
c. osteoblasts
d. macrophages
e. thrombocytes

53. Which type of connective tissue has the most fluid in its matrix?
a. bone
b. ligaments
c. blood
d. muscle
e. adipose

54. The dermis of the skin is made of what type of tissue?
a. hemopoietic tissue
b. blood
c. cartilage
d. dense regular connective tissue
e. dense irregular collagenous

55. Arterial walls consist of what type of tissue?

a. hemopoietic tissue

b. dense irregular elastic

c. reticular

d. dense regular connective tissue

e. all of the above

56. Lymph nodes will contain what type of tissue?

a. hemopoietic tissue

b. reticular tissue

c. cartilage

d. dense regular connective tissue

e. none of the above

57. The disks found between the bodies of the vertebrae are what type of tissue?

a. hyaline cartilage

b. elastic cartilage

c. fibrocartilage

d. loose connective tissue

e. dense connective tissue

58. What muscle type of voluntary?

a. skeletal

b. cardiac

c. smooth

59. What muscle type of the makes up about 40% of our body weight?

a. skeletal

b. cardiac

c. smooth

60. What muscle type of found only in the heart?

a. skeletal
b. cardiac
c. smooth

61. What muscle type makes up much of the digestive tract?
a. skeletal
b. cardiac
c. smooth

62. What muscle type is multinucleated and has nuclei at the edges of the cell?
a. skeletal
b. cardiac
c. smooth

CHAPTER 5 – Answers to multiple choice questions.

1. B
2. B
3. E
4. E
5. A
6. A
7. A
8. B
9. C
10. A
11. B
12. A
13. D
14. B
15. A
16. C
17. A
18. C
19. D
20. B
21. A
22. C
23. A
24. B
25. E
26. A
27. B
28. A
29. C
30. B

31. B
32. E
33. A
34. B
35. C
36. A
37. B
38. A
39. C
40. E
41. D
42. D
43. C
44. A
45. A
46. C
47. B
48. B
49. E
50. B
51. A
52. B
53. C
54. E
55. B
56. B
57. C
58. A
59. A
60. B
61. C
62. A

Human Skin Diagram

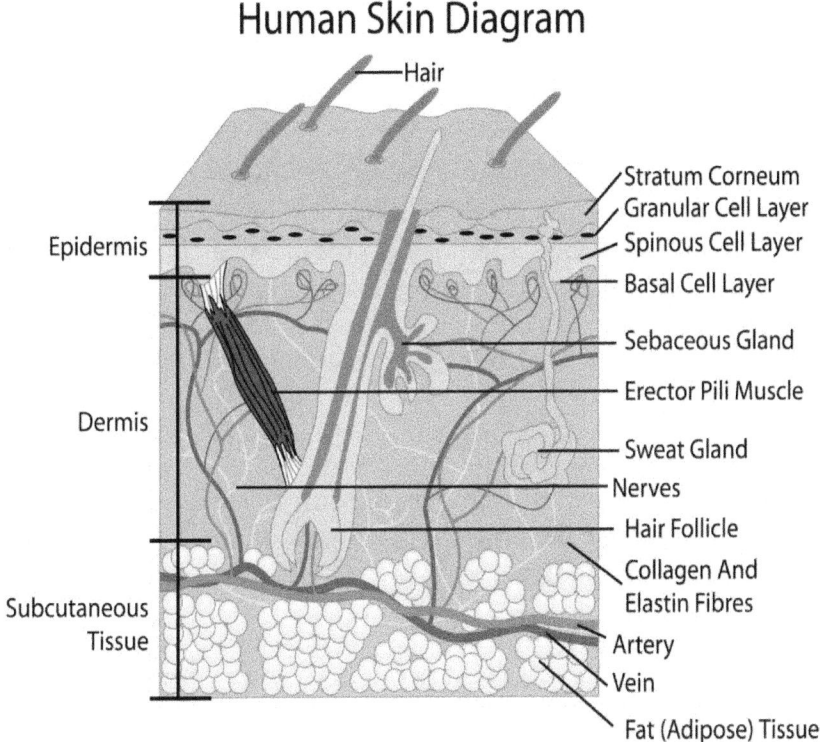

Hair

Epidermis

Dermis

Subcutaneous Tissue

Stratum Corneum
Granular Cell Layer
Spinous Cell Layer
Basal Cell Layer
Sebaceous Gland
Erector Pili Muscle
Sweat Gland
Nerves
Hair Follicle
Collagen And Elastin Fibres
Artery
Vein
Fat (Adipose) Tissue

CHAPTER 6

Integumentary System

The integumentary system includes not just our skin, but also hair, nails and some glands of the body. The glands are those which are superficial and found in your skin. Some of these glands everyone has heard of.

Functions of integumentary system

Some of the functions of this system are easy to see. Most people will think of protection, when they think of the integumentary system. Largely what our skin does is provide a barrier around our body. Don't think of the skin as only keeping things out, because it also keeps many things in our body. If someone loses a large amount of skin, they will also lose large amounts of fluids and can become dehydrated.

Our skin contains countless numbers of sensory receptors in it also. Many of the senses we are consciously aware of are associated with the skin (touch, itch, pain, etc.).

Our skin has a great deal to do with our body temperature. Everyone knows when we get hot, we sweat. This sweating will help cool the body. When we get cold, we shiver. Shivering heats up the body. Something else to consider is vasodilation and vasoconstriction of the blood vessels in the dermis. Think of the blood vessels in your skin, as being like the radiator in a car. When your engine heats up, water is pumped through the radiator to release heat. When we heat up we dilate the blood vessels in our skin to get heat release. It is cooler at the surface of our body, so when we bring more blood there, we release more het. When we get cold, we see blood vessels doing the opposite, they will constrict in our skin. As we keep blood deeper in the body, we conserve heat.

The skin is part of our immune system, because it does keep foreign invaders out of our body.

A small amount of waste removal is associated with the skin, but it is minor. Vitamin D production begins in our skin also.

Students often get confused with the layers found within this system. The breakdown is:

Integumentary system has 2 layers: epidermis and dermis. Don't forget the hypodermis is not part of this system.

1. Epidermis - The outer layer, this is stratified squamous epithelial tissue.

2. Dermis – The deeper layer and where all the strength of our skin is, because this is where the collagen and other fibers are found. Most all structures of the skin are found in this layer.

The epidermis has 5 layers (strata) with in it:

1. Stratum basale – The deepest layer, where mitosis is occurring to replace the outermost layers, which are always being lost. Melanocytes can be found at this layer.

2. Stratum spinosum – The second layer on our way up the strata. This layer gets its name, because the cells can look spiny as they try to separate on the way up.

3. Stratum granulosum – This middle layer gets its name because the cells look very dark and grainy on prepared slides. When epithelial cells reach this layer, they are mostly dead, start to change from a cuboidal to squamous shape, and have many materials added to them like keratin and melanin.

4. Stratum lucidum – This is a layer which will only be found in thick skin areas of the body. Thick skin areas are the palms of our hands and the bottom of our feet. These areas are under more stress and abrasion, so our body has an extra layer within it for more protection.

5. Stratum corneum – This layer is the most superficial, the one you see on the surface of your skin. This layer is by far the thickest stratum of the epidermis and it is even thicker in the thick skin areas.

The epidermis gives us a great deal of protection. The melanin within it protects us from ultraviolet light. Everyone knows of the damage the UV rays of the sun can cause. The keratin within these cells makes a good barrier and that is what this layer is for. Melanin gives color to our skin, hair and to the iris of the eye.

The epidermis doesn't have blood vessels penetrating it. Avascular is one characteristic of epithelial tissues. Why don't we want blood vessels to penetrate this layer? The blood would be too close to the surface of the body. Blood would be lost easily and foreign materials could get into it easily.

Most of the cells seen in the epidermis are of the keratinocyte type. Getting there name from the protein they produce (keratin). Keratin helps to make these cells into a strong barrier. Some cells will be melanocytes. Getting there name from melanin, the material protecting us from UV radiation.

Desquamation – The process by which the outer layer of epithelial cells are always falling away and being replaced by new cells. This process helps to keep foreign materials off of our skin.

Keratinization – The process by which keratin and other materials are added to epithelial cells as they make their way up the strata.

Consider how and why our skin changes color. It gets red when more blood flows through it, this will occur when we are hot or feeling strong emotions. It may get pale or bluish, when blood is restricted from it. It grows darker when more melanin is produced within it.

GLANDS

1. lactiferous (milk) glands-mammary glands

2. ceruminous (earwax) glands

3. sebaceous (oil) glands – produce oily material called sebum

- lubricates hair and causes skin to repel water

4. sweat glands

a. merocrine – most common

- temp sensitive, evaporative cooling

b. apocrine – secrete water and acids

- pungent body odor

The dermis has 2 layers: papillary and reticular.

1. Papillary layer – The superficial layer of the dermis. This layer is very thin and gives us our fingerprints and footprints. The layer will push up on the epidermis creating ridges. These ridges give us more friction when we hold objects with our hands. It also gives traction for the bottom of our feet.

2. Reticular layer – This deeper layer of the dermis is by far the thickest and the strongest layer. Many collagen fibers are found here and they are always there for strength. Most all of the structures in the skin are found in this layer.

Stretch marks (striae) occur in the body when the dermis is being stretched, faster than it can grow. Even though we see stretch marks in the epidermis, stretch marks have nothing to do with it.

Arrector pili muscles will be found in the dermis and will stand a hair up, when the muscle is told to contract by the nervous system. This action gives us a barrier between the skin and outside environment, when we get cold.

Hypodermis (subcutaneous tissue)

This layer is not part of the integumentary system. Don't forget that, it will probably be a test question. You will know when you get into this deep layer when you see all of the adipocytes. This is a fatty layer, which holds heat in our body and also acts as a cushion for deeper structures. About half the fat in our body is in this layer, so we have this padding.

Other cells will include macrophages to stop the entry of foreign invaders and fibroblasts to build fibers.

Hair

Hairs are places where the epidermis penetrates deep and produces these bound cells. A hair has three main sections to it: shaft (part above the surface), root (part beneath the surface) and bulb (deep, round section where the hair grows from).

Nails

Nails are places where our epithelial cells grow stronger. We get many functions from our nails. They will protect the ends of our digits, help in defense, to dig, etc.

A nail has the following anatomy:

-nail body – nail itself

-free edge – part you clip

-cuticle (eponychium) – proximal portion of nail

- nail root – area where nail is generated, deep

- lunula – white, crescent shape area

- hyponychium – region under free edge

- nail groove – sides of nail, holds in place

- nail fold – ridge over groove, holds in place

Burns

Burns come in three different types or degrees.

1st degree – When the epidermis is damaged and redness is seen.

2nd degree – When the epidermis and dermis are damaged, blisters will be seen.

3rd degree – When both layers of the skin are destroyed and gone.

QUESTIONS

1. What structures are found in the integumentary system?

2. What layers make up the skin?

3. What is the dominant fiber of the dermis?

4. What is the function of melanin?

5. Name the types of glands in the integumentary system and describe the function of each.

Chapter 6 – Questions

1. How many layers are found in the integumentary system?
a. 1
b. 2
c. 3
d. 4
e. 5

2. Which of the following layers is not part of the integumentary system?
a. epidermis
b. dermis
c. hypodermis
d. reticular layer
e. papillary layer

3. How many layers (strata) are found in the epidermis of the skin?
a. 1
b. 2
c. 3
d. 4
e. 5

4. How many layers are found in the dermis of the skin?
a. 1
b. 2
c. 3
d. 4
e. 5

5. What are the two primary layers found in the integumentary system?
a. papillary and epidermis
b. epidermis and dermis
c. dermis and reticular
d. papillary and reticular
e. dermis and hypodermis

6. What are the two layers of the dermis?
a. papillary and epidermis
b. epidermis and dermis
c. dermis and reticular
d. papillary and reticular
e. dermis and hypodermis

7. What is the name of the skin layer you can see on the surface of your skin?
a. epidermis
b. dermis
c. hypodermis
d. reticular layer
e. papillary layer

8. What is the name of the deepest layer of the epidermis?
a. stratum corneum
b. stratum lucidum
c. stratum granulosum
d. stratum spinosum
e. stratum basale

9. Which of the following is not found in the integumentary system?
a. skin
b. hair

c. nails

d. glands

e. teeth

10. Which gland is associated with cooling the body?

a. sweat

b. sebaceous

c. ceruminous

d. sweat and sebaceous

e. all of the above

11. Which gland will secrete oil onto the skin?

a. sweat

b. sebaceous

c. ceruminous

d. sweat and sebaceous

e. all of the above

12. Which gland can be found in the ear producing wax?

a. sweat

b. sebaceous

c. ceruminous

d. sweat and sebaceous

e. all of the above

13. How would you describe the epidermis?

a. simple squamous

b. stratified cuboidal

c. pseudostratified

d. stratified squamous

e. transitional

14. What vitamin is produced partially in the skin?

a. A
b. B
c. C
d. D
e. E

15. Most cells of the epidermis will be producing what material?
a. melanin
b. keratin
c. sebum
d. water
e. lipids

16. What material in the skin protects us from ultraviolet light?
a. melanin
b. keratin
c. sebum
d. water
e. lipids

17. In what layer of the epidermis does mitosis occur?
a. stratum corneum
b. stratum lucidum
c. stratum granulosum
d. stratum spinosum
e. stratum basale

18. Which epidermis layer is only found in thick skin areas?
a. stratum corneum
b. stratum lucidum
c. stratum granulosum
d. stratum spinosum
e. stratum basale

19. Which epidermis layer is the thickest?
a. stratum corneum
b. stratum lucidum
c. stratum granulosum
d. stratum spinosum
e. stratum basale

20. Which layer of the dermis is the most superficial?
a. epidermis
b. dermis
c. hypodermis
d. reticular layer
e. papillary layer

21. Which layer of the dermis is the thickest and contains most of the structures?
a. epidermis
b. dermis
c. hypodermis
d. reticular layer
e. papillary layer

22. Which layer of the dermis gives us fingerprints and footprints?
a. epidermis
b. dermis
c. hypodermis
d. reticular layer
e. papillary layer

23. What fiber provides most of the strength of the skin?
a. collagen
b. reticular

c. elastic

24. Sebum is secreted by which gland?
a. sweat
b. sebaceous
c. ceruminous
d. sweat and sebaceous
e. all of the above

25. What part of a hair is seen above the surface of the skin?
a. shaft
b. root
c. bulb
d. medulla
e. cortex

26. What burn will have blisters?
a. first degree
b. second degree
c. third degree

CHAPTER 6 – Answers to multiple choice questions.

1. B
2. C
3. E
4. B
5. B
6. D
7. A
8. E
9. E
10. A
11. B
12. C
13. D
14. D
15. B
16. A
17. E
18. B
19. A
20. E
21. D
22. E
23. A
24. B
25. A
26. B

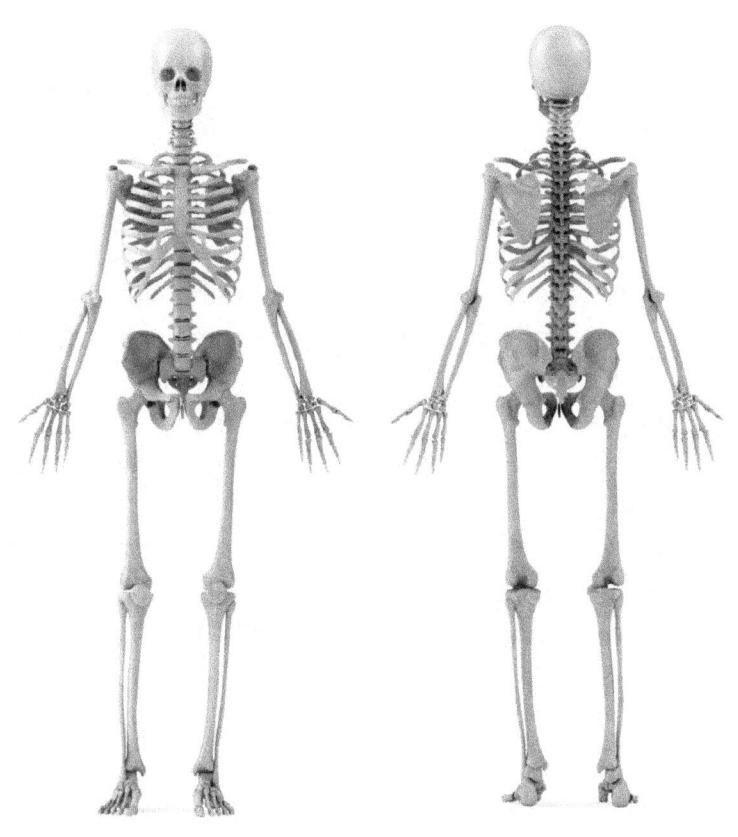

CHAPTER 7 – Skeletal System

The average human has 206 bones in their body. You would think that we would all have the same number of bones, but it is common to see a deviation in the number. Some people have extra bones in the skull, extra vertebrae, ribs, etc.

Functions of skeletal system

1. Protection of deeper organs.   With bone being the strongest tissue in our body, we use it to protect other structures in us. The skull protects the brain, sternum and ribs protect the heart and lungs, etc.

2. Supporting our bodies.   Bones are like the steel and concrete inside of a building. This framework is what all of the other structures are attached to in one way or another. Our overall appearance is due to the presence of our bones.

3. Movement of our bodies.   Most of what we think of as movement is the use of our skeletal muscles pulling on our bones. Our muscles use our bones as simple levers to accomplish what we need of them.

4. Storage. Our bones store many materials for future use. We could all name calcium as a stored material, but energy is stored in fat cells, phosphates are stored in the hard mineral part of bone and other materials.

5. Hematopoiesis. This is a fancy way of saying, "Creation of the cells in our blood." Every cell we see in our blood was made in our red bone marrow. Red bone marrow is also called hematopoietic tissue.

Structures in the skeletal system

1. Bone tissue makes up most of the skeletal system. We will cover the contents of this tissue soon.

2. Ligaments are the dense regular collagen arrangements which bind our bones together.

3. Cartilage is very much involved with the skeletal system. We will see cartilage almost everywhere we see bones.

 Hyaline cartilage will be found covering bones at a joint. Wherever bones come together you want this hard, smooth, glassy cartilage in between them to reduce friction. Where you see bones growing and developing early in our lives, you will also find hyaline cartilage there.

Fibrocartilage pads will be found in some joints, acting as shock absorbers. This prevents bones from slamming together and causing damage. Intervertebral disks between our vertebrae, meniscus in our knees and cushions in jaws are all places we find fibrocartilage. Cartilage will grow from within (interstitial growth) or on the surface (appositional growth). You will only see appositional growth with bones. Bones are too hard to expand, so they won't grow from within, only at the surface.

Bone shapes
Bones can be found in our body in 4 basic shapes.
1. Short bones. Short bones will actually look square, rectangular or round. The carpals in our wrists and the tarsals in our ankles are good examples of these bones.
2. Long bones. Longs bones must be long and cylinder shaped. This category can be confusing. Some bones like sternum and ribs look like they should be long bones, but they are considered flat bones, because they are thin and flat. Don't be surprised if sternum or rib shape is on an exam. Long bones are seen in the upper and lower limbs. Long bone anatomy will include the terms:
-Diaphysis – the long, straight part of the bone.
-Epiphysis – the odd shaped end pieces of the bone.
-Epiphyseal plate – the area toward the end of a long bone, where the bone gets longer. This zone of cartilage will change into a hard bone plate called the epiphyseal line in adulthood.
-Medullary cavity – the hollow space to the center, where we find red bone marrow.
3. Flat bones. Flat bones will always be thin. The large bones of the skull, like the frontal, parietal, temporal and occipital bones are good examples.

4. Irregular bones. If any bone won't easily fit into one of the previous categories or it has a crazy shape, it will belong to this group. Vertebrae and sphenoid bones are good examples.

Bone tissue. We need to know what is in bone.
Bone tissue will contain three big cell types: osteoblasts (bone builders), osteoclasts (break down bone) and osteocytes (maintain bone-build a little). We learned these suffixes in a previous chapter, so don't forget them. Don't confuse bone tissue with a bone, these are two different structures. A bone is an organ, since it contains bone tissue and red bone marrow. Bone tissue is a collection of cells and matrix. This will sometimes be a test question. Osteoblasts and osteoclasts will always be found on the outside of bone and osteocytes will always be found deeper in the bone, living inside of a small space called a lacunae. Radiating off of these lacunae will be many tiny cracks called canaliculi.

Our bones are always changing (remodeling) to adapt to the stresses, we put on them. This remodeling process is the result of osteoblast and osteoclast activity. If our bones are to remain healthy we need vitamin D, calcium, vitamin C (collagen synthesis) and other materials.

In any tissue you don't just have the cells, but also the matrix. The matrix of bone is made largely of two materials: collagen and hydroxyapatite (bone salt).
The collagen is in the bone to give bone flexibility. We don't think of our bones as being flexible, but they are, if they are healthy. Now remember a collagen fiber won't stretch, but it will bend, just like a steel cable. This is where the flexibility comes from. This material makes about 1/3 of the bone matrix.

The hydroxyapatite is the hard mineral part of the bone. This is where the strong weight bearing strength of bone comes from. This material makes about 2/3 of the bone matrix.

To understand why we have these two materials in bones, compare bone construction to bridge construction. Think of what a bridge looks like when it is partially completed. Looking inside the bridge you see two materials: steel bars and concrete. Why are the steel bars in the bridge? For flexibility. If you are standing on a bridge when a car goes over it, you can feel the bridge move (this is the flexibility). Why is the concrete in the bridge? To give it weight bearing strength (to hold the cars weight).

What would happen if the bridge was built entirely from steel bars? It would be too flexible. Our bones are too flexible if we don't have enough of the hard materials in them. Someone with bowed legs didn't have enough hydroxyapatite in their bones at some time. The lower limbs bowed under the weight of the body, because they were too flexible.

What would happen if the bridge was built entirely from concrete? It would not be flexible enough. The bridge would soon crack and break, as it was used. Without enough collagen in our bones, they will crack and break easily. A lack of collagen is one thing that causes brittle bones in the elderly.

Bone structure
You will see many times of bones in your text, here are a few:
1. Compact bone – This is the type of bone you usually see in slides, where you see what looks like tree stumps. This is the very dense, hard bone type seen superficially around bones.

2. Cancellous (spongy) bone – This is hard bone tissue, but there are lots of spaces in between the structures called trabeculae. Anytime you see trabeculae, you think cancellous bone, because that is where you find it. This bone is not soft, it only looked like a sponge to someone. The trabeculae connect in all directions giving strength the deeper regions of bones. It is often found in the ends of bones also.

3. Woven bone (immature bone) – This is young, new bone.

4. Lamellar bone (mature bone) – Developed bone.

5. You still have your different bone shapes also.

Blood calcium

We all know that we have calcium in our bones. It is there for strength in the hydroxyapatite, but it's also there for storage. Bone is a connective tissue and one of the functions of bone, is storage. Think about why we have osteoclasts. When would we want to break down bone? We want to store calcium and later release it, to balance our blood calcium levels. We need proper levels of calcium in our body for other functions such as: clotting, muscle contraction and membrane potentials.

To balance calcium in our blood and body, we have two hormones for doing this.

1. Calcitonin – This hormone will inhibit osteoclasts in our bones. If we inhibit osteoclasts, we are stopping the release of calcium. We want to stop calcium release, when we have adequate amounts of calcium in our blood. This hormone is released when calcium levels are adequate or high.

2. Parathyroid hormone (PTH) – This hormone will stimulate osteoclasts in our bones. If we stimulate osteoclasts, we release calcium from the bones. Remember, materials are delivered to

tissues by the blood, so if we break the tissue back down, the materials go back into the blood. So, stimulating osteoclasts will release calcium from the bones and help to raise our blood calcium levels. PTH also targets other tissues.

The small intestine is targeted and PTH will tell the small intestine cells to absorb calcium as it passes through the GI tract. This will also raise our blood calcium levels.

The kidneys are also targeted and PTH will tell the kidneys to reabsorb calcium back into our body. This will raise blood calcium levels.

PTH will also increase vitamin D production. Vitamin D will increase calcium absorption in the small intestine. All of this will raise blood calcium levels, so PTH is released when blood calcium levels are low. This is a simple negative feedback mechanism.

Development of Bone
Bones develop in two major ways.

1. Intramembranous ossification – This is a type of bone development seen before we are born and in the first two years of life. Only a few of our bones develop by this process and they are mostly in the skull. The flat bones of the skull are good examples of where this type of ossification is found. This type of bone development originates from tissue other than cartilage. This tissue is not as rigid as cartilage and this gives flexibility to the head at the time of birth. The soft spots in the skull between these developing bones are what we call soft spots (fontanels).

2. Endochondral ossification – This type of bone development involves hyaline cartilage. Most bones of our body were hyaline cartilage before they were bone. Bone growth will always start at the center of a bone (primary ossification centers) and the new bone will develop on the outside of the old bone (appositional growth). Towards the ends of long bones we will see a zone of this cartilage and it's at this spot, we see long bones getting longer. This cartilage

zone (epiphyseal plate) is where our long bones, get longer. As we reach maturity this epiphyseal plate (cartilage) will change into the epiphyseal line (bone), at this time we reach our maximum height. Some of the original hyaline cartilage remains on the bone and covers the ends of them at joints. This cartilage will make a hard, glassy cover to reduce friction.

Our skeletal system is divided into 2 big divisions:
1. Axial division – These are the bones down the center of the body. Skull, hyoid, vertebrae, ribs and sternum.
2. Appendicular division – The bones of our upper and lower limbs, plus the pectoral and pelvic girdles (the bones which hold our upper and lower limbs to the axial division).

Some facts about the skeletal system
1. 206 bones for most people.
2. 80 bones in the axial division.
3. 126 bones in the appendicular division.
4. 22 bones in the skull.
5. 26 bones in the adult vertebral column. 7 cervical, 12 thoracic, 5 lumbar, 1 coccygeal
6. Paranasal sinuses are the bones with hollow spaces, which lead into the nasal cavity. These bones are frontal, maxillary, sphenoid and ethmoid. These hollow spaces lighten the skull and affect our speech.
7. Average adult has 32 teeth. 8 incisors, 4 canine, 8 premolar and 12 molars.
8. 12 pairs (24) ribs. Pairs 1-7 are true ribs, 8-12 are false ribs and 11-12 are also floating ribs.
9. The lateral bone in your forearm is the radius.
Your text will have many pictures of bones. Good luck, lots of memorization.

ARTICULATIONS – Joints

An articulation is just a fancy way of saying joint. A joint is anywhere two or more bones come together.

You need to be familiar with the major types of joints in the body. I will be as brief as possible about each.

The structural classification is the most widely used. There are 3 structural classifications with a few subcategories under them.

1. Fibrous joint – A joint bound together by collagen fibers. This joint has little to no movement in between the bones.

  Three subcategories.

   a. syndesmoses – A joint bound by ligaments.

   b. gomphoses – A joint found between the teeth and alveolar processes.

   c. sutures – The joints between the flat bones of the skull.

2. Cartilaginous joint – A joint bound by cartilage, hyaline or fibrocartilage only.

   a. synchondroses - A joint bound by hyaline cartilage.

   b. symphyses – A joint bound by fibrocartilage.

3. Synovial joint – A more complex joint, which is surrounded by a fluid filled cavity called a bursa.

   a. hinge joint – A round cylinder surrounded by a C-shaped structure. Like the hinge of a door. Example - elbow

   b. saddle joint – Joint shaped like a saddle for a horse. Example – base of your thumb.

   c. pivot joint – Joint where a bone turns on its long axis. Example – the turning of the radius when you rotate your hand.

   d. ellipsoid joint – Take a ball and socket joint and change it into a football like shape. Example – where the first cervical vertebrae meets the skull.

e. ball and socket joint – Simply a ball shape resting in a hollow socket. Example – shoulder and hip.

f. gliding joint – Two flat opposing surfaces sliding over each other. Example – facets of the vertebrae.

MOVEMENTS of joints

1. Flexion – to bend or decrease the angle between bones. One exception is at the knee.

2. Extension - to straighten or increase the angle between bones. One exception is at the knee.

3. Elevation – to move a body part in a superior direction.

4. Depression – to move a body part in an inferior direction.

5. Plantar flexion – to stand on your toes.

6. Dorsiflexion – to go back on your heels.

7. Abduction – to move a body part away from the midline of the body.

8. Adduction – to move a body part towards the midline of the body.

9. Rotation – to turn a body part on its long axis. Think of spinning a pipe.

10. Pronation – to turn the palm down or to lie face down.

11. Supination – to turn the palm up or to lie on your back.

12. Circumduction – to move in a circular, cone shape motion. Can only be done at the hip and shoulder, where we have ball and socket joints.

13. Protraction – to glide forward in the anterior direction.

14. Retraction – to glide back in a posterior direction.

15. Lateral Excursion - move the mandible right or left.

16. Medial Excursion – return the mandible to the center.

17. Inversion – to turn the bottom of your foot in.

18. Eversion – to turn the bottom of your foot out.

QUESTIONS

1. What are the major functions of the skeletal system?

2. How many bones does the average adult have?

3. What is the difference between the axial and appendicular skeleton?

4. How many bones are found in the human skull?

5. Which has more bones in it, the axial or appendicular skeleton?

6. What 2 materials make up bone and each should make up what percentage of bone?

7. What are the 3 cell types found in bone?

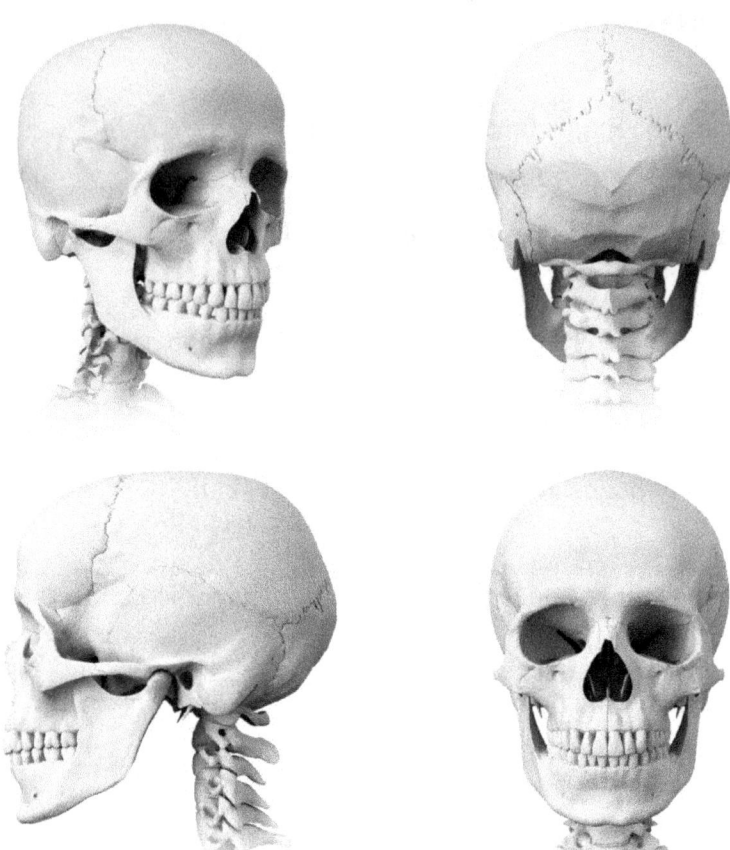

Chapter 7 – Questions

1. The average human has how many bones in the body?

a. 125

b. 106

c. 200

d. 206

e. 254

2. Which of the following is not a function of the skeletal system?

a. hematopoiesis

b. storage

c. protecting deeper structures

d. supporting the body

e. vitamin D production

3. What structures bind bone to bone?

a. ligaments

b. tendon

c. reticular fibers

d. elastic fibers

e. dermis

4. The humerus would be which bone shape?

a. short

b. long

c. flat

d. irregular

e. none of the above

5. Thoracic vertebrae would be which bone shape?

a. short

b. long

c. flat

d. irregular

e. none of the above

6. Which cell type is responsible for bone growth?

a. osteoblast

b. osteoclast

c. osteocyte

d. canaliculi

e. osteons

7. Which cell type is responsible for maintaining bone tissue?

a. osteoblast

b. osteoclast

c. osteocyte

d. canaliculi

e. osteons

8. Which cell type is responsible for calcium release from bone?

a. osteoblast

b. osteoclast

c. osteocyte

d. canaliculi

e. osteons

9. Most bones develop from what type of cartilage?

a. hyaline

b. fibrocartilage

c. elastic cartilage

10. What type of cartilage can be found covering the ends of bones, providing a smooth, glassy surface?

a. hyaline

b. fibrocartilage

c. elastic cartilage

11. What type of cartilage can be found in between the bodies of the vertebrae acting as a cushion?

a. hyaline

b. fibrocartilage

c. elastic cartilage

12. What fiber is found in abundance in bone matrix?

a. collagen

b. elastic

c. reticular

13. What fiber gives our bones flexibility?

a. collagen

b. elastic

c. reticular

14. What is the name of the hard, mineral material found in the matrix of bone?

a. osteons

b. canaliculi

c. haversian system

d. hydroxyapatite

e. trabeculae

15. After an osteoblast has surrounded itself with bone matrix it becomes an (a)?

a. osteoclast

b. osteocyte

c. osteoclast

d. dead cell

e. red blood cell

16. What vitamin is needed for calcium absorption?

a. A

b. B

c. C

d. D

e. E

17. What vitamin is needed for collagen production?

a. A

b. B

c. C

d. D

e. E

18. Which hormone decreases osteoclast activity?

a. calcitonin

b. parathyroid hormone

c. vitamin D

d. vitamin E

e. hydroxyapatite

19. Parathyroid hormone will do which of the following?

a. increase osteoclast activity

b. increase vitamin D production

c. increase calcium absorption in the small intestine

d. increase calcium reabsorption in the kidneys

e. all of the above

20. Which hormone works to increase blood calcium levels?

a. calcitonin

b. parathyroid hormone

c. vitamin D

d. vitamin E

e. hydroxyapatite

21. Which hormone works to decrease blood calcium levels?

a. calcitonin

b. parathyroid hormone

c. vitamin D

d. vitamin E

e. hydroxyapatite

22. Most bones develop by what process?

a. intramembranous ossification

b. endochondral ossification

23. Which bone is found in the axial division of the skeletal system?
a. humerus
b. radius
c. pubis
d. femur
e. vertebrae

24. Which bone is found in the appendicular division of the skeletal system?
a. rib
b. sternum
c. hyoid
d. carpal
e. xyphoid process

25. How many bones are found in the average human skull?
a. 14
b. 22
c. 24
d. 30
e. 41

26. How many cervical vertebrae does the average human have?
a. 7
b. 12
c. 5
d. 1
e. 9

27. How many vertebrae does the average adult have?
a. 12

b. 21

c. 26

d. 30

e. 31

28. Which bone of the forearm is lateral (remember the anatomic position)?

a. carpal

b. radius

c. ulna

d. humerus

e. metacarpal

29. The tarsal bones are found where?

a. wrist

b. ankle

c. neck

d. lower back

e. skull

30. The largest bone in the body is?

a. femur

b. humerus

c. coxal bones

d. tibia

e. fibula

31. The average adult has how many teeth?

a. 20

b. 24

c. 30

d. 32

e. 38

32. The first 7 pairs of ribs are called?

a. true ribs

b. false ribs

c. floating ribs

33. How many ribs does the average human have?

a. 12

b. 20

c. 24

d. 30

e. 32

34. How would you identify a cervical vertebra?

a. It has an extra set of facets.

b. It has a large, heavy body.

c. It has 3 holes in it.

d. The spinous process points down sharply.

e. none of the above

35. The sacrum is a fusing of how many bones during embryonic development?

a. 2

b. 4

c. 5

d. 6

e. 8

36. What part of a vertebrae is the most anterior?

a. body

b. spinous process

c. transverse process

d. vertebral foramen

e. vertebral arch

37. How many bones are found in the axial division of the skeleton?
a. 126
b. 80
c. 206
d. 94
e. 156

38. The bones of the fingers and toes are?
a. carpals
b. metacarpals
c. phalanx bones
d. tarsals
e. metatarsals

39. Hallux is another name for what?
a. index finger
b. nose
c. big toe
d. pelvis
e. lower limb

40. A joint bound together by collagen fibers is?
a. fibrous joint
b. cartilaginous joint
c. synovial joint
d. saddle joint
e. gliding joint

41. The peg and socket joints where teeth fit into alveolar processes are which joint?
a. gomphoses

b. suture

c. synovial joint

d. ellipsoid joint

e. symphyses

42. Osteocytes live inside hollow spaces in bone called?

a. canaliculi

b. osteons

c. lacunae

d. lamellae

e. central canal

43. In the center of each osteon is a hole called?

a. canaliculi

b. osteons

c. lacunae

d. lamellae

e. central canal

44. Longs bones get longer at what region?

a. diaphysis

b. epiphysis

c. medullary cavity

d. epiphyseal plate

e. articular cartilage

45. The frontal and parietal bones have what shape?

a. short

b. long

c. flat

d. irregular

e. none of the above

46. The soft spots found on a baby's skull are called?
a. epiphyseal plates
b. fontanels
c. lacunae
d. central canals
e. osteons

47. Shrugging your shoulders is an example of what action?
a. flexion
b. elevation
c. dorsiflexion
d. protraction
e. inversion

48. Bending your arm at your elbow is an example of what action?
a. flexion
b. elevation
c. dorsiflexion
d. protraction
e. inversion

49. Placing your weight back on your heels is an example of what action?
a. flexion
b. dorsiflexion
c. plantar flexion
d. pronation
e. supination

50. Going up on your toes is an example of what action?
a. flexion
b. dorsiflexion
c. plantar flexion

d. pronation
e. supination

CHAPTER 7 – Answers to multiple choice questions.

1. D
2. E
3. A
4. B
5. D
6. A
7. C
8. B
9. A
10. A
11. B
12. A
13. A
14. D
15. B
16. D
17. C
18. A
19. E
20. B
21. A
22. B
23. E
24. D
25. B
26. A
27. C
28. B
29. B
30. A
31. D

32. A
33. C
34. C
35. C
36. A
37. B
38. C
39. C
40. A
41. A
42. C
43. E
44. D
45. C
46. B
47. B
48. A
49. B
50. C

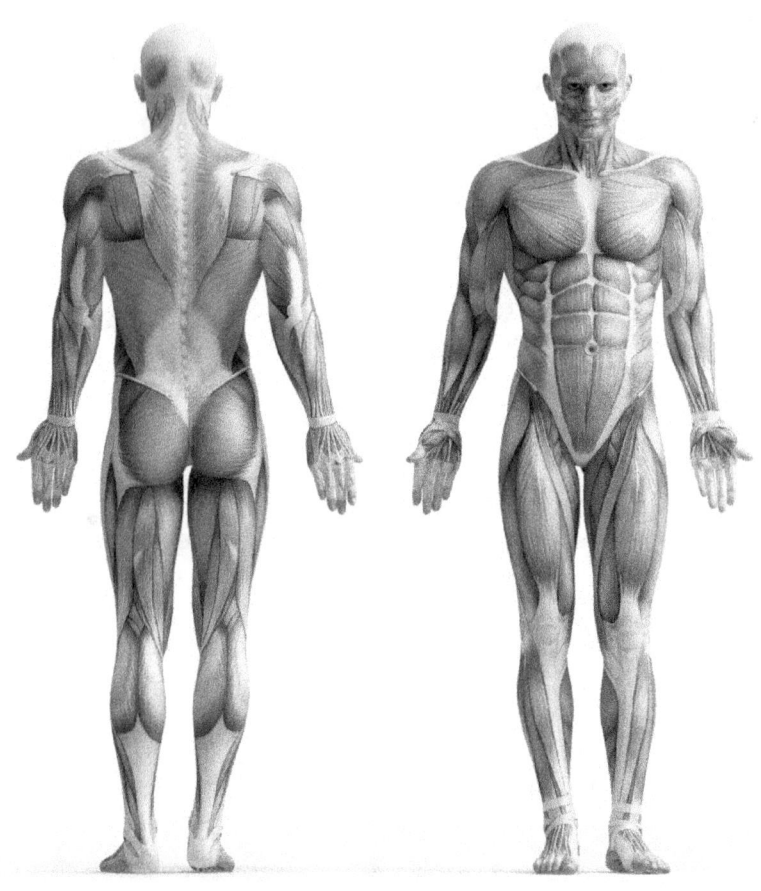

CHAPTER 8 – Muscular System

Muscles are used in the body for one general purpose, they get shorter and this causes them to pull on things. Muscles do have many functions, but it all comes down to their ability to contract (get shorter). We will take a muscle down to the chemical level and see how it contracts.

Muscles have the characteristic of being excitable. This means they are capable of responding to signals from the nervous and endocrine system.

Extensibility is the ability of a muscle to return to its original length after contraction.

We have seen in a previous chapter that we have three types of muscles in our body. Usually when someone says, "muscle", they are speaking of skeletal muscle. All three types of muscle are very similar in how they work, but they do have small differences. We will concentrate on skeletal muscle and speak more about cardiac and smooth in future chapters.

Comparison of Muscle types
1. Skeletal and cardiac have a cylinder shape. Smooth muscle has a spindle shape. This means it's thick in the center and tapered at the ends, like a football.
2. Cardiac and smooth have one nucleus, centrally located. Skeletal is multinucleated and the nucleus is at the periphery (outer edge). Skeletal muscle cells originate from several smaller cells during embryonic development. These muscle building cells are called myoblasts. Myo means muscle in Latin and blast cells build.
3. Each has a different function. Skeletal muscle is attached to bones and obviously pulls on them. Cardiac muscle is only found in the heart and generates blood pressure. Smooth muscle is found in many places and has many functions.
4. Cardiac and smooth muscle are involuntary (work automatically), but skeletal is consciously controlled.
5. Skeletal and cardiac muscle are striated (have stripes), smooth doesn't.

You will be asked at least one question over the similarities and differences of the muscle types.

You also need to know some general terminology, which is used with muscles.

1. Tendon – A dense collagen arrangement binding a bone to a muscle.
2. Origin (head) – The more stationary end of attachment of a muscle.
3. Insertion – The more movable end of attachment of a muscle. When a muscle contracts, you will notice that one end of the muscle doesn't move (origin) and the other does (insertion).
4. Action – The movement accomplished by a muscle.
5. Endomysium – The connective tissue surrounding each muscle cell.
6. Epimysium – The connective tissue surrounding an entire muscle.
7. Perimysium – The connective tissue surrounding fasciculi (bundles of muscle cells).
8. Aponeurosis – A broad, flat tendon. Most of tendons are cable like in appearance.
9. Synergists – A group of muscles working together to accomplish the same action.
10. Agonist – The muscle responsible for a particular action. A muscle opposed by another.
11. Antagonist – A muscle opposing an agonist.
12. Fixators – Muscles used to strengthen and stabilize a joint.
13. Sarcoplasm – The cytoplasm of a muscle cell.
14. Sarcolemma – The plasma membrane of a muscle cell.
15. Sarcoplasmic reticulum – The smooth endoplasmic reticulum of a muscle cell. This structure stores up large amounts of calcium, which is needed for muscle contraction.
16. Sarcomere – The region between two Z disks.

17. Z disks – The attachment sites for actin myofilaments.

18. Troponin – Structure calcium binds to during muscle contraction.

19. Motor neuron – a neuron controlling muscle cells.

20. Motor unit – One motor neuron and the group of muscle cells it innervates.

21. All or None Principle – When applied to muscle, this principle tells us this. When a muscle cell contracts it always does it with the same amount of force every time. A muscle cell can't contract a little or a lot; it either does or it doesn't, with no in between. Notice this applies to a muscle cell and not an entire muscle. A muscle applies additional force by recruiting more motor units. When you lift something light, you only use a few motor units within a muscle. When you lift something heavy you are using many motor units within a muscle.

22. Tetany – Muscle contraction without relaxation.

23. Acetylcholine – A neurotransmitter used by a motor neuron to open ligand gated sodium channels on skeletal muscle.

24. Aerobic respiration – ATP building process requiring oxygen. This process is what supplies most energy to cells, including muscle.

25. Rigor mortis – The stiffening of muscles seen in a person after death. The absence of ATP and the presence of calcium cause this stiffening.

26. Slow muscle fibers – Myofilaments which contract slowly. This type of filament will work for long periods of time and be fatigue resistant. These have a well-developed blood supply and are found in red meats.

27. Fast muscle fibers – Myofilaments which contract rapidly. This type of filament will work for short periods of time and fatigue quickly. These have a poorly developed blood supply and are found in white meats.

28. Anaerobic respiration – An energy building process, which takes place in the absence of oxygen. Lactic acid is a waste byproduct from this process.

29. Treppe – An increase in muscle contraction strength seen as a muscle contracts several times after a resting period. This increase in strength is caused by the presence of increasing calcium quantities.

30. Atrophy – A loss in size of muscle or muscle cells.

31. Hypertrophy – An increase in size of a muscle or muscle cells.

3 classes of Levers

Our skeletal muscles get their name, because they are attached to the skeletal system. When we want to move our body, we use the nervous system to contract these muscles and pull on bones. Our bones are used as simple levers, similar to what we see with tools.

With all classes of levers three variables will be found in each: fulcrum, weight and pull.

The muscle will be providing the pull, the bone will act as the lever and the fulcrum is the pivot point (joint). You will see these three variables used in each lever, but notice they won't be in the same arrangement in the three classes.

1. Class 1 lever – A lever where the fulcrum (pivot point) is between the weight and the pull. Think of a see saw, when you think of this lever. Children alternate going up and down, but the pivot point remains in the center. You will see this type of lever in the body, when a person looks up and down. The head moves forward and back, but the pivot point over the cervical vertebrae remains in the center.

2. Class 2 lever – A lever where the weight is in between the fulcrum and the pull. Think of a wheel barrow, when you lift on the handles, your upper limbs provide the pull. The fulcrum (pivot

point) is way out over the wheel and the weight you want moved is in the center. You see this lever used when we go up on our toes. The pull comes from the gastrocnemius and soleus muscles on the posterior side of our leg and we pivot out over our toes. The weight of our body is in between the two, resting over our tibia.

3. Class 3 lever – A lever where the pull is in between the weight and the fulcrum. This is the most common type of lever in the body. When you use a shovel the weight you want moved is out in the broad part of the shovel and your hand on the handle is the fulcrum. Your other hand provides the pull in between the two. When we flex our biceps brachii muscle, the muscle is pulling in between the other two.

Remember these 3 classes, an example of a tool that works in a similar way and a place in the body where you see the lever at work.

Muscle anatomy
You will need to know the anatomy of a muscle all the way down to the chemical level. The six levels of a muscle cell from largest to smallest are:
1. Muscle – This is the entire muscle, which is composed of many muscle fasciculi (cell bundles).
2. Fasciculi – These are bundles of muscle cells.
3. Muscle cell – Your author will probably call these muscle fibers. That is a common nickname since the cells are long and cylinder shaped.
4. Myofibrils – Bundles of muscle filaments inside of a muscle cell.
5. Sarcomeres – The region of a myofibril found between two Z disks.
6. Myofilaments – The two types of myofilaments are actin and myosin. These two proteins are where muscle contraction is

occurring. We will look closer at them, when going over the steps involved in muscle contraction.

NEUROMUSCULAR JUNCTION

What happens at the neuromuscular junction? Know these steps.

1. An action potential is conducted down the end of an axon.
2. This action potential opens voltage gated calcium channels near the axon terminal.
3. The influx of calcium causes vesicles of acetylcholine to move to the edge of the synapse.
4. Acetylcholine is released by exocytosis into the synapse.
5. Acetylcholine diffuses across the synapse and binds to ligand gated sodium channels on the skeletal muscle cell.
6. Sodium enters the skeletal muscle cell.
7. The influx of sodium generates an action potential on the plasma membrane of the muscle cell.
8. The enzyme acetylcholinesterase breaks down acetylcholine and removes it from the ligand gated sodium channels.
9. Choline is brought back up into the axon and recycled.

What happens after the neuromuscular junction? The steps following the events at the neuromuscular junction are what's called, "Excitation – Contraction." This next series of steps covers what happens with the muscle cell after the events of the neuromuscular junction.

1. We left off above with the following: An action potential has been generated on the plasma membrane of the skeletal muscle.
2. The action potential will be brought deep within the cell by the transverse tubules (T-tubules).
3. Along the T-tubules is sarcoplasmic reticulum (smooth endoplasmic reticulum). As the action potential travels along the sarcoplasmic reticulum, it will open up voltage gated calcium channels.

4. Voltage gated calcium channels on the sarcoplasmic reticulum open.
5. Calcium leaves the sarcoplasmic reticulum and enters the environment around the actin and myosin.
6. Calcium binds to troponin.
7. Troponin moves the tropomyosin, exposing the active sites on the actin filaments.
8. Myosin heads bind to the active sites on the actin myofilaments. This is called cross bridge formation.
9. Myosin breaks down ATP.
10. Myosin flexes at the hinge region, pulling the actin myofilaments closer together.
11. ATP replaces the ADP on the myosin, causing it to release from the actin.
12. As long as ATP and calcium are present, the muscle will continue to contract.

Smooth muscle
2 types are found in the human body.
a. Single unit – This type of smooth muscle works together in a very coordinated fashion. The muscle cells have many gap junctions between them. The gap junctions allow for good communication between the cells and the better cells communicate the better they work together.

b. Multiunit – These muscle cells have fewer gap junctions, so they don't communicate as well. With less communication the cells work more independently.

Cardiac muscle
Remember that cardiac muscle is only found in the heart. This muscle is used to generate the pressure to move blood around the

body. Intercalated disks are communication structures only found in the heart, so don't forget these.

Chapter 8 – Questions

1. Which muscle has a spindle shape?
a. skeletal
b. cardiac
c. smooth

2. Which muscle has a nucleus at the periphery (outer edge)?
a. skeletal
b. cardiac
c. smooth

3. Which muscle is voluntary?
a. skeletal
b. cardiac
c. smooth

4. Which muscle doesn't have striations?
a. skeletal
b. cardiac
c. smooth

5. Which muscle is found in more locations than the others?
a. skeletal
b. cardiac
c. smooth

6. Which muscle makes 40% of our body weight?
a. skeletal
b. cardiac
c. smooth

7. Which muscle is found only in the heart?

a. skeletal

b. cardiac

c. smooth

8. What is the name of a structure that binds bone to muscle?

a. tendon

b. ligament

c. perimysium

d. sarcomere

e. fixator

9. A muscle has two ends of attachment. Which is the more stationary end of attachment?

a. agonist

b. antagonist

c. origin (head)

d. insertion

e. troponin

10. A muscle has two ends of attachment. Which is the more movable end?

a. agonist

b. antagonist

c. origin (head)

d. insertion

e. troponin

11. The movement accomplished by a muscle is?

a. agonist

b. antagonist

c. action

d. insertion

e. aponeurosis

12. A group of muscles working together?
a. synergists
b. antagonists
c. action
d. fixators
e. motor units

13. Muscles used to strengthen and stabilize a joint?
a. synergists
b. antagonists
c. action
d. fixators
e. motor units

14. The plasma membrane of a muscle cell?
a. sarcolemma
b. sarcomere
c. Z disk
d. troponin
e. sarcoplasm

15. The structures responsible for storing calcium inside of muscles?
a. sarcoplasm
b. sarcolemma
c. sarcoplasmic reticulum
d. sarcomere
e. fixators

16. The region between two Z disks?
a. sarcoplasm

b. sarcolemma

c. sarcoplasmic reticulum

d. sarcomere

e. fixators

17. What does calcium bind to inside of a skeletal muscle during muscle contraction?

a. agonist

b. antagonist

c. origin (head)

d. insertion

e. troponin

18. What neurotransmitter is released into the synapse between a neuron and a skeletal muscle?

a. norepinephrine

b. epinephrine

c. acetylcholine

d. serotonin

e. none of the above

19. Skeletal muscles obtain most of their energy from?

a. anaerobic respiration

b aerobic respiration

20. Which lever class is the most common?

a. class 1

b. class 2

c. class 3

21. Which lever class works like a see saw?

a. class 1

b. class 2

c. class 3

22. Which lever class works like a wheel barrow?
a. class 1
b. class 2
c. class 3

23. Which lever class has the pull in the middle?
a. class 1
b. class 2
c. class 3

24. Flexing at your elbow is an example of which lever class?
a. class 1
b. class 2
c. class 3

25. What type of smooth muscle has many gap junctions?
a. single unit
b. multi-unit

26. Which of the following is caused by smooth muscle?
a. walking
b. swallowing
c. movement in the stomach
d. pressure in the heart
e. talking

27. An increase in muscle size is?
a. vasoconstriction
b. atrophy
c. synergy
d. treppe

e. hypertrophy

28. The myofilament with the active site located on it?
a. actin
b. myosin
c. sarcomere
d. sarcoplasm
e. sarcolemma

29. A muscle contains many bundles of muscle cells called?
a. fasciculi
b. myofibrils
c. myofilaments
d. sarcomeres
e. none of the above

30. Action potentials are brought deep inside a skeletal muscle by?
a. myofilaments
b. sarcoplasmic reticulum
c. T tubules
d. troponin
e. Z disks

31. Which of the following filaments gets shorter during muscle contraction?
a. actin
b. myosin
c. both
d. neither

32. When an action potential is sent through a muscle what happens?
a. the muscle dies

b. the muscle contracts

c. the muscle relaxes

33. Acetylcholine opens what ion channels on skeletal muscle?

a. potassium

b. calcium

c. chloride

d. sodium

e. magnesium

34. The space between the neuron and the muscle cell is?

a. troponin

b. synapse

c. Z disks

d. sarcomeres

e. myofibril

35. What type of ion channels does acetylcholine bind to?

a. nongated

b. ligand gated

c. voltage gated

d. leak channels

36. What ion provides most of the positive charge on the outside of a cell?

a. potassium

b. calcium

c. chloride

d. sodium

e. magnesium

37. Without acetylcholine a muscle would never?

a. contract

b. relax

38. Without acetylcholinesterase a muscle would never?
a. contract
b. relax

39. When myosin binds to actin this is called?
a. cross bridge formation
b. excitation
c. treppe
d. rigor mortis
e. inhibition

40. ATP is needed for?
a. muscle contraction
b. muscle relaxation
c. neither
d. both

41. A circular muscle will always?
a. flex a structure
b. extend a structure
c. abduct a structure
d. elevate a structure
e. close something

42. What muscles rotate the head?
a. trapezius
b. pectoralis major
c. temporalis
d. masseter
e. sternocleidomastoid

43. The pectoral major muscles are used when doing what?
a. sit ups
b. standing
c. pushups
d. rowing
e. opening your eyes

44. The latissimus dorsi muscles are used when?
a. sit ups
b. standing
c. pushups
d. rowing
e. opening your eyes

45. Which muscles are used to close the eyes?
a. zygomaticus major
b. masseter
c. temporalis
d. orbicularis oculi
e. frontalis

46. The temporalis muscles are used for?
a. chewing
b. seeing
c. sneezing
d. coughing
e. none of the above

47. Which muscle is used for flexing at the elbow?
a. rectus femoris
b. biceps brachii
c. triceps brachii
d. rectus femoris

e. tibialis anterior

48. The quadriceps femoris muscles are used for
a. sit ups
b. standing
c. pushups
d. rowing
e. opening your eyes

49. The longest muscle in the body is?
a. rectus femoris
b. sartorius
c. gastrocnemius
d. pectoralis major
e. latissimus dorsi

50. Flexing at the knees is the result of what muscles?
a. quadriceps femoris
b. hamstrings
c. rectus femoris
d. gastrocnemius
e. tibialis anterior

51. Standing on your toes is accomplished by using what muscles?
a. quadriceps femoris
b. hamstrings
c. rectus femoris
d. gastrocnemius
e. tibialis anterior

52. The muscles on the anterior surface of the forearm are?
a. flexors
b. extensors

c. fixators

d. originators

e. supinators

53. Dimples are found in what muscles?

a. buccinators

b. zygomaticus

c. temporalis

d. mentalis

e. orbicularis oris

54. The primary muscle of ventilation is?

a. internal intercostals

b. diaphragm

c. rectus femoris

d. internal oblique

e. deltoid

55. Needles are commonly injected into what muscles?

a. trapezius

b. pectoralis major

c. gluteus medius

d. gluteus maximus

e. teres minor

CHAPTER 8 – Answers to multiple choice questions.

1. C
2. A
3. A
4. C
5. C
6. A
7. B
8. A
9. C
10. D
11. C
12. A
13. D
14. A
15. C
16. D
17. E
18. C
19. B
20. C
21. A
22. B
23. C
24. C
25. A
26. C
27. E
28. A
29. A
30. C

31. D
32. B
33. D
34. B
35. B
36. D
37. A
38. B
39. A
40. D
41. E
42. E
43. C
44. D
45. D
46. A
47. B
48. B
49. B
50. B
51. D
52. A
53. D
54. B
55. C

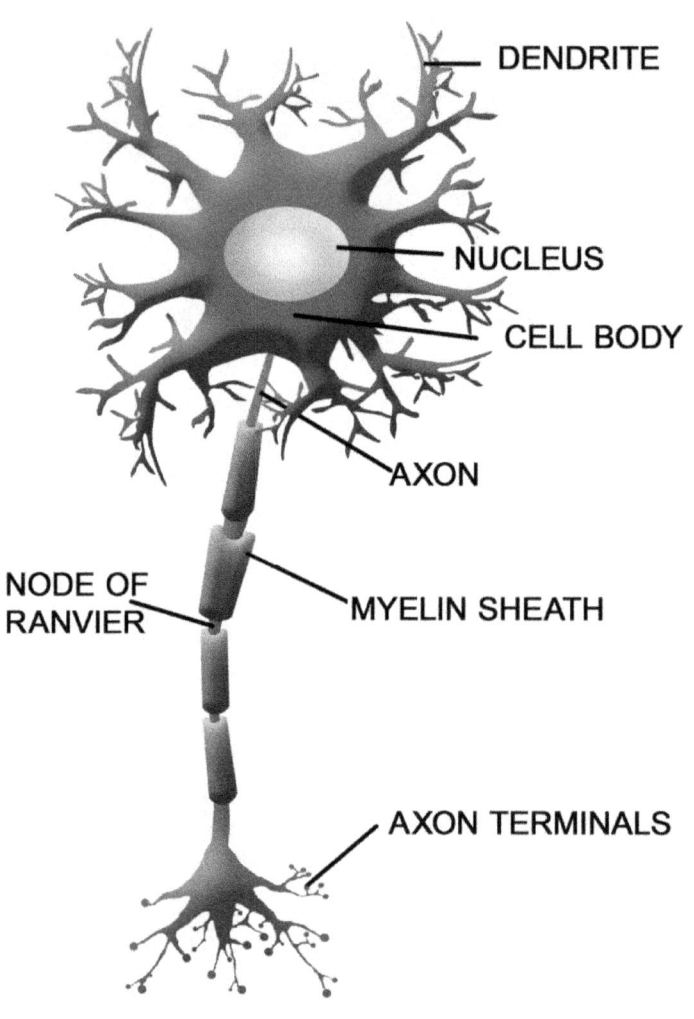

DENDRITE

NUCLEUS

CELL BODY

AXON

NODE OF
RANVIER

MYELIN SHEATH

AXON TERMINALS

CHAPTER 9 – Nervous System

The first thing you need to know about the nervous system are the different divisions. Make sure you know the divisions and what is in each one of them.

Divisions of the Nervous System

CNS – central nervous system – brain and spinal cord

PNS – peripheral nervous system – nerves, sensory receptors, ganglia

> -Sensory division – all signals coming in to the CNS
> - Motor division – all signals going out from the CNS
> > -Somatic – outgoing signals for control of skeletal muscle
> > -Autonomic – outgoing signals to all else. Controls involuntary functions.
> > > -Sympathetic – fight or flight division. Prepares for physical activity.
> > > -Parasympathetic division – rest and relaxation division
> > > -Enteric – local control of digestive system

Neurons can be classified in many ways, one way is based on their function. The direction of the action potential and where it is going, is what is different about these neurons.

Functional classification of Neurons
1. Sensory neurons (afferent neurons) – incoming signals. Any neuron which sends an action potential towards the spinal cord or brain is a sensory neuron.
2. Motor neurons (Efferent) – outgoing signals. Any neuron which sends an action potential away from the spinal cord or brain is a sensory neuron.
3. Interneurons – in between a sensory and motor.

Another way to classify neurons is based on the structure. The only thing different about these neurons is the number of dendrites. Pay careful attention to the number of dendrites in each. It is easy to confuse them.

Structural classification of Neurons
1. Multipolar neurons – many dendrites and one axon.
2. Bipolar neurons – one dendrite and one axon. Called bipolar since it has one dendrite (one pole) and one axon (another pole).
3. Unipolar neurons – no dendrites and one axon.

The nervous system is occupied by two types of cells, neurons and neuroglial cells (all other cells in the nervous system). Neurons take up about half of the nervous system and the neuroglial cells take up the other half. Neuroglial cells, also called glial cells, are supporting cells of the nervous system. These cells are supporting the neurons. Glial cells will help neurons to survive and perform their jobs properly.

Neuroglial Cells of the Central Nervous System
1. Astrocytes – epithelial cells making the blood brain barrier. Allow for nutrient and waste exchange. Astrocytes surround the capillaries in the brain. Since they surround these capillaries, these cells can determine what can leave the blood and enter the brain. These cells are here to protect the brain from harmful chemicals and foreign invaders. This very special barrier is present to protect the neurons, because if the neurons are lost, they won't be replaced.

2. Ependymal cells – epithelial cells lining the ventricles of the brain. Produce cerebrospinal fluid. The ventricles are the four fluid filled cavities deep inside the brain. This fluid provides nutrients to the neurons and makes a fluid cushion around the brain and spinal cord. The cilia on the cell surface are there to move the fluid through the ventricles.

3. Microglial – white blood cells of the nervous system. These cells will remove anything which doesn't belong (foreign invaders, chemicals, dead cells, etc.)

4. Oligodendrocytes – form myelin sheaths around axons. Act as insulation for action potentials. The insulation around the axon is like rubber around a copper wire in an electrical appliance. The insulation keeps the electricity in the wire and our axons need the same insulation. Another function of the myelin is to speed up action potentials.

Neuroglial Cells of the Peripheral Nervous System
1. Schwann cells – form myelin sheaths around axons. These cells provide the myelin insulation in the peripheral nervous system. Myelin always keeps the action potentials in the axon and speeds up the action potential.

2. Satellite cells – surround the bodies of neurons to help provide nutrients. Neurons are the most active cells in the body, so they require large amounts of nutrients to function properly.

Membrane Potentials
Understanding the electric charges in cells is important to any understanding of how a neuron works. Make sure you understand where the electric charges come from, how they are produced and what they are used for.
Let's study action potentials by answering the following questions.
1. What is the resting membrane potential?
The electric charge found on a cell membrane when the cell is at rest. When the cell is at rest the outside (extracellular charge) will be positive and the inside (intracellular charge) will be negative.
2. Where does the resting membrane potential come from?
The charges come from charged particles called ions. The cell will put more of the positive ions (cations) on the outside of the cell and it will put more of the negative ions (anions) on the inside of the cell. Sodium and calcium are found in high concentrations on the outside of the cell and the sodium provides the greatest amount of the

positive charge. Potassium is found mostly on the inside of the cell, even though it has a positive charge. The inner negative charge comes mostly from proteins and phosphate ions.

3. What sets up these charges?

The resting membrane potential is established primarily by the sodium potassium exchange pump. This pump is a protein found in the plasma membrane and is the best example of active transport in the body. Every time this pump consumes an ATP molecule, it moves 3 sodium out of the cell and 2 potassium in to it. The sodium is trapped outside until something (chemical or electric signal) opens the gates and lets it in. After the potassium is pulled into the cell, much of it will diffuse back out of the cell through nongated ion channels.

4. What is it called when the charges on the cell swap position? In other words, when the inside becomes positive, instead of the outside.

This is called depolarization when the charges swap. Most depolarization is the result of sodium movement into the cell.

5. What happens when the charges swap?

When the charges swap position an action potential is generated.

6. What is an action potential?

An action potential is an electric signal generated by a cell.

7. What is it called when the charges return to the resting state? In other words, when the outside charge becomes positive again.

This is called repolarization of the cell.

8. What do cells use action potentials for?

Action potentials are used for cellular communication. Neurons use electric and chemical signals to communicate with the cells of our body. One of the advantages of an electric signal is that it travels very fast. So they can be used when rapid communication is needed.

Action potentials are often described as propagating. This means that they move. When an action potential is generated down an axon, one action potential doesn't move all the way down an axon. It generates an electric signal, which will generate another action potential beside it. This second action potential will generate a third and so on. So many different action potentials travel down an axon or on a cell membrane, not one. This is what is meant by the action potential propagation, the generation of one action potential after another.

Saltatory conduction is the jumping of the action potentials between the myelin sheaths. If myelin didn't have gaps in between them (nodes) then action potentials would travel much slower. Think of how a grass hopper can move. He can walk (moves slowly) or he can hop (moves fast). The jumping of electric signals from one gap (node) to the next, speeds them up. As we get older and lose the myelin, our action potentials can no longer jump, so they slow down.

QUESTIONS
1. What are neuroglial cells?

2. What are neurons?

3. What is myelin?

Cells of the Central Nervous System

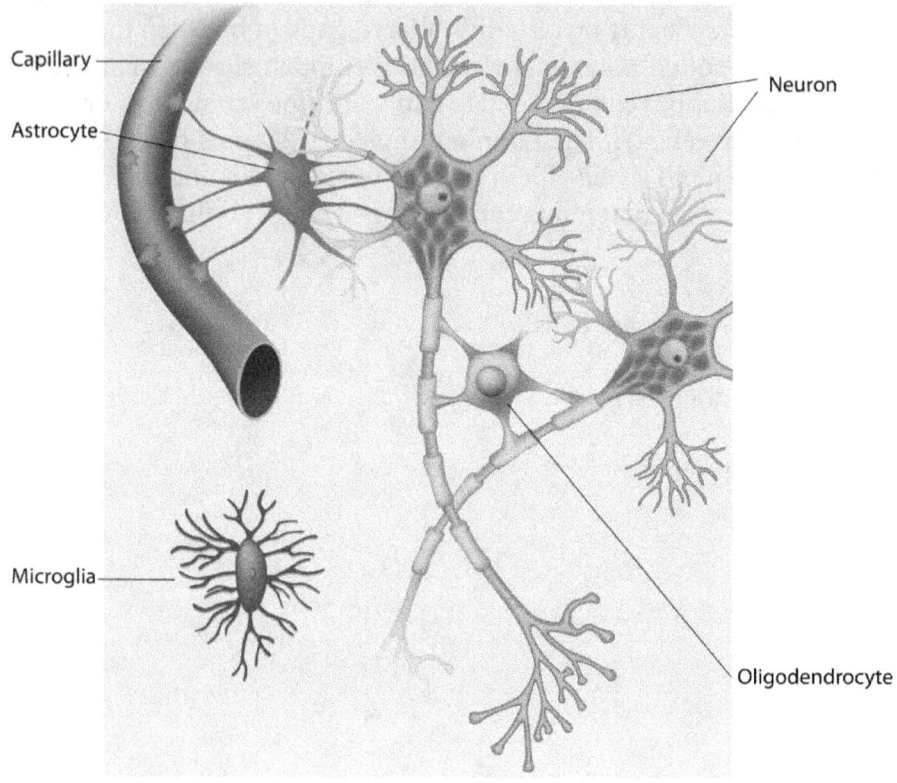

Capillary

Astrocyte

Microglia

Neuron

Oligodendrocyte

Chapter 9 – Questions

1. What division of the nervous system contains the brain?
a. central nervous system
b. peripheral nervous system
c. sensory division
d. motor division
e. autonomic division

2. What division of the nervous system contains the spinal cord?
a. central nervous system
b. peripheral nervous system
c. sensory division
d. motor division
e. autonomic division

3. What division of the nervous system prepares the body for physical activity?
a. sympathetic
b. somatic
c. enteric
d. sensory
e. motor

4. What division of the nervous system controls automatic functions of the body?
a. central nervous system
b. peripheral nervous system
c. sensory division
d. motor division
e. autonomic division

5. A neuron with one dendrite would be a?
a. multipolar neuron
b. bipolar neuron
c. unipolar neuron

6. A neuron with many dendrites would be a?
a. multipolar neuron
b. bipolar neuron
c. unipolar neuron

7. A neuron with no dendrites would be a?
a. multipolar neuron
b. bipolar neuron
c. unipolar neuron

8. A sensory neuron is also called a (an)
a. afferent neuron
b. efferent neuron
c. bipolar neuron
d. interneuron
e. none of the above

9. A neuron conducting its electric signal towards the central nervous system would be a?
a. motor neuron
b. interneuron
c. sensory neuron

10. A neuron conducting its electric signal away from the central nervous system would be a?
a. motor neuron
b. interneuron
c. sensory neuron

11. Which of the following cells is not found in the central nervous system?
a. astrocyte
b. ependymal
c. microglial
d. oligodendrocyte
e. schwann

12. Which cell forms the blood brain barrier?
a. astrocyte
b. ependymal
c. microglial
d. oligodendrocyte
e. schwann

13. Which cell produces cerebrospinal fluid?
a. astrocyte
b. ependymal
c. microglial
d. oligodendrocyte
e. schwann

14. Which cell will remove and destroy foreign substances in the nervous system?
a. astrocyte
b. ependymal
c. microglial
d. oligodendrocyte
e. schwann

15. Which of the following cells produces myelin in the central nervous system?

a. astrocyte
b. ependymal
c. microglial
d. oligodendrocyte
e. schwann

16. Which cell will provide nutrients to the neurons?
a. satellite
b. ependymal
c. microglial
d. oligodendrocyte
e. schwann

17. What is an action potential?
a. chemical signal
b. electric signal
c. temperature signal
d. mechanical signal
e. unknown signal

18. What ion is primarily responsible for the resting membrane potential?
a. calcium
b. potassium
c. sodium
d. chloride
e. magnesium

19. When the cell membrane is positive on the outside and negative on the inside, this is called?
a. depolarized
b. resting membrane potential
c. negatively charged

d. positively charged

20. When the cell membrane becomes positive on the inside, this is called?
a. depolarized
b. resting membrane potential
c. negatively charged
d. positively charged

21. A neuron will send a signal out to another cell through what structure?
a. dendrite
b. axon
c. cell body
d. schwann cell
e. satellite cell

22. A neuron will receive signals through what structures?
a. dendrite
b. axon
c. cell body
d. schwann cell
e. satellite cell

23. A neuron found between a sensory and motor neuron is?
a. motor neuron
b. interneuron
c. sensory neuron

24. A rapid movement of sodium from the outside of the cell to the inside would cause?
a. depolarization
b. repolarization

c. hyperpolarization

d. hypopolarization

25. When the charge on a cell membrane becomes greater in difference than what it was before, this is called?

a. depolarization

b. repolarization

c. hyperpolarization

d. hypopolarization

26. When the charge on a cell membrane becomes less in difference than what it was before, this is called?

a. depolarization

b. repolarization

c. hyperpolarization

d. hypopolarization

27. The space between two neurons is called the?

a. ligand

b. terminal

c. synapse

d. vesicle

e. none of the above

28. A nerve is a collection of many?

a. schwann cells

b. cell bodies

c. dendrites

d. axons

e. astrocytes

CHAPTER 9 – Answers to multiple choice questions.

1. A
2. A
3. A
4. E
5. B
6. A
7. C
8. A
9. C
10. A
11. E
12. A
13. B
14. C
15. D
16. A
17. B
18. C
19. B
20. A
21. B
22. A
23. B
24. A
25. C
26. D
27. C
28. D

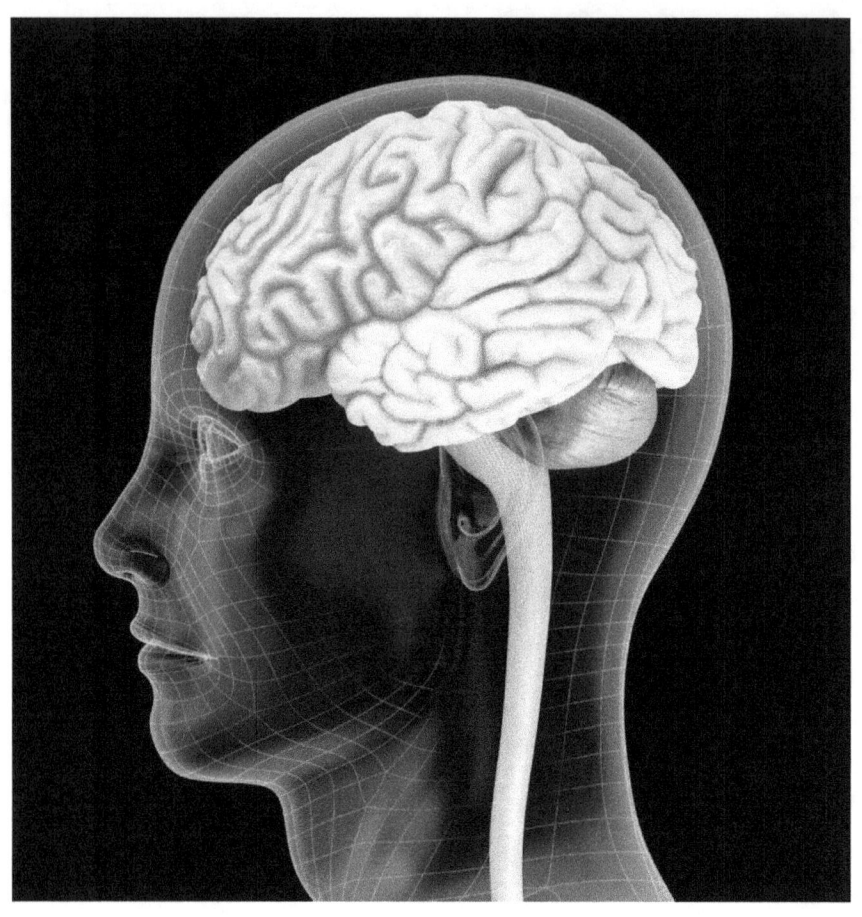

CHAPTER 10 - Brain

The brain has 4 major regions, make sure you are familiar with them.

Cerebrum, cerebellum, brainstem, diencephalon

1. Cerebrum – largest part of brain. This is where we have our consciousness, memory and emotions. The cerebrum forms the bulk of the brain and covers the brain on all but the inferior surface. The cerebrum is separated into two halves called hemispheres. These two hemispheres are separated by a deep fissure called the longitudinal fissure. This deep fissure separates the two hemispheres down to the corpus callosum, where axons cross over from one side of the brain to the other.

So there is a left and right hemisphere. Each one of the hemispheres is divided into four lobes (sometimes five). These lobes are named the same as the flat bones of the skull, which are directly superficial to them. The lobes are frontal, parietal, occipital and temporal. Separating the frontal and parietal lobes is a depression called the central sulcus. This groove can be seen laterally on both sides of the brain.

The surface of the cerebrum is very wavy and this is what gives it an odd appearance. The wavy surface increases surface area, making room for more neurons and axons. Any groove on the surface of the brain is called a sulci. Think of the sulci as sucked in areas. Any elevation on the brain is called a gyri. Think of these as the elevated areas between the sulci.

Inside the brain two areas can be seen with nothing but the eyes. This material is white matter and grey matter. White matter is the region where the myelin and the axons are found. Grey matter is the region where the dendrites and the neuron cell bodies are found. These regions can be seen in spinal cord also, but the grey matter of the spinal cord is deep, where the grey matter of brain is superficial.

Major functions of the cerebral lobes are:
Frontal – voluntary motor function
Parietal – sensory perception
Occipital – vision
Temporal - hearing

2. Cerebellum – small part of brain found deep to occipital bone. The primary function of the cerebellum is learning complex movements of the skeletal muscles.

   The major regions of the cerebellum include two large lateral hemispheres, two small floculonodular lobes and the vermis in the center. On the outer surface of the cerebellum many ridges called folia can be seen. They look like thick stacks of paper. On the inside of the cerebellum is a mylineated area called the arbor vitae. This area looks like a tree to the inside.

3. Diencephalon – deep center of the brain. If the brain is cut in half, a midsaggital view will show the diencephalon region deep in the center. This deep region, just inferior to the corpus callosum, has four regions to it. Each one of these regions has the name thalamus in its name.
a. The thalamus is where most all sensations pass. This region receives sensations before they pass on to the cerebrum. Smell is the only sensation which doesn't pass through the thalamus.
b. The hypothalamus is an area with many important functions, necessary for life. Some of these functions are the satiety center (hunger center), thirst center, temperature regulation, many endocrine functions and more. The hypothalamus is the part of the brain which regulates the pituitary gland. This gland produces more major hormones than any other part of the body.
c. subthalamus – found beneath the thalamus.
d. epithalamus – posterior region of diencephalon. The pineal gland is in this area. The pineal gland will regulate yearly sleep/wake cycles and control the onset of puberty.

4. Brainstem – the inferior part which connects brain to spinal cord. The brainstem ends around the foramen magnum, which is where the spinal cord begins. The brainstem has 3 sections and they are listed from superior to inferior.
Midbrain – superior portion. The superior colliculi give us visual reflexes. When you are driving down the road and a rock hits your wind shield, you quickly move your head. The neurons in this

region are connected to your vision and if anything comes at your eyes rapidly, the superior colliculi contract the muscles in your neck. This movement will protect your face.

The inferior colliculi give us auditory reflexes in a similar way. If something loud startles you, you tend to jump away from the noise.

Pons – center section. Helps to regulate ventilation.

Medulla oblongata – inferior section, contains nuclei vital to survival. This part of the brainstem contains neurons which regulate vital functions, such as cardiac and respiratory functions. Damage to the medulla oblongata usually means death. The pyramids and olives work together to coordinate muscular activity for balance.

The brain has 3 Meninges – connective tissues surrounding the brain and spinal cord. Make sure you know these tissues in order from superficial to deep.

a. Dura mater (meningeal dura) – thickest, most superficial layer. Found just deep to the bones surrounding the brain.

b. Arachnoid mater – middle of the layers, fibers in this connective tissue looked like a spider web to someone so that is where it received its name.

c. pia mater – deepest layer, bound tightly to the surface of the brain.

Ventricles

The ventricles are four fluid filled cavities located deep within the brain. Ependymal cells cover the inside of these chambers and produce this fluid. Cerebrospinal fluid is produced at the choroid plexus. Here fluid and nutrients are removed and cilia move the fluid through the chambers. Most of the fluid is produced in the two large lateral ventricles. From here the fluid travels through the interventricular foramen to the third ventricle. From here the fluid travels down the cerebral aquaduct to the fourth ventricle at the base of the cerebellum.

Cranial nerves

12 pairs of cranial nerves can be seen on the inferior surface of the brain. Make sure you know the functions of these nerves.

Cranial nerves and functions

1. Olfactory – sense of smell.

2. Optic – vision

3. Oculomotor – Moves four of the six muscles which move our eyes. It also opens our eyes, controls the size of our pupils and the lens. Specific muscles controlled are:

Four muscles which move our eyes - inferior rectus, medial rectus, superior rectus, inferior oblique. The levator palpebrae superioris which opens our eyes. The smooth muscle of the pupil which regulates how much light enters our eyes. The ciliary muscle of the lens for focusing on objects near and far.

4. Trochlear – Controls one of the six muscles which move our eyes. The muscle is the superior oblique.

5. Trigeminal – Sensory to the face and forehead. Controls the muscles involved with chewing (mastication). The chewing muscles are the masseter, temporalis, lateral pterygoids and medial pterygoids.

6. Abducent – Controls the last eye muscle the lateral rectus.

7. Facial – Controls most of the facial muscles. Some taste from the tongue, two pairs of salivary glands and lacrimal glands (tear glands).

8. Vestibulocochlear – hearing and balance.

9. Glossopharyngeal – some taste, one pair of salivary glands and throat muscles (swallowing).

10. Vagus – nerve connections to almost everything in the thoracic and abdominal cavities.

11. Accessory – controls the trapezius and sternocleidomastoid muscles.

12. Hypoglossal – controls tongue and throat muscles.

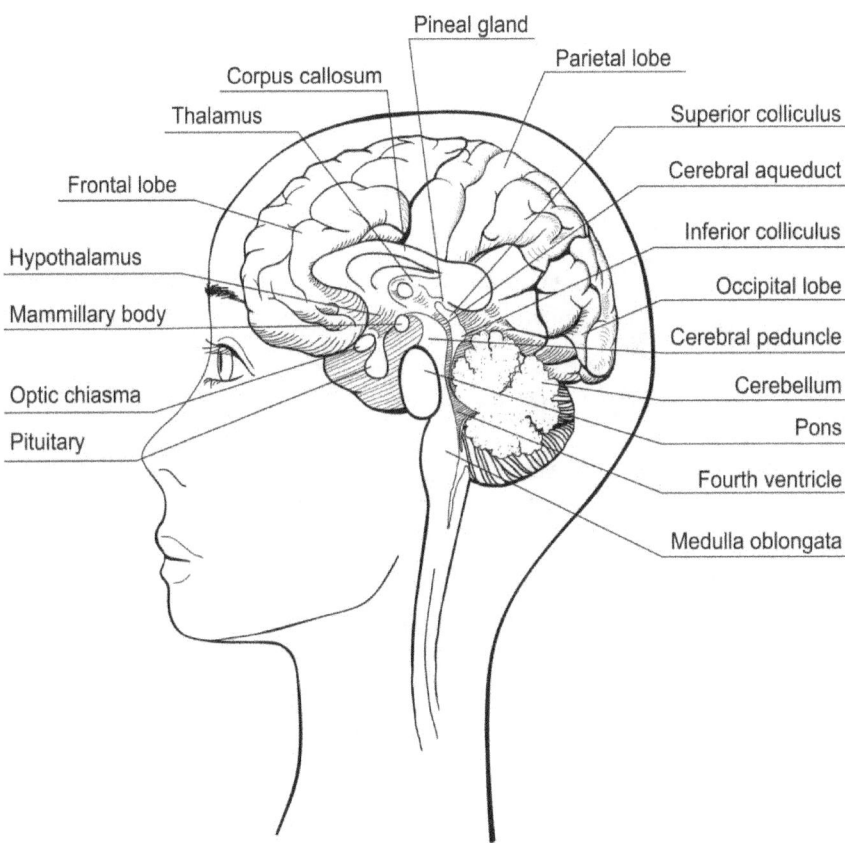

Pineal gland

Corpus callosum

Parietal lobe

Thalamus

Superior colliculus

Frontal lobe

Cerebral aqueduct

Inferior colliculus

Hypothalamus

Occipital lobe

Mammillary body

Cerebral peduncle

Cerebellum

Optic chiasma

Pons

Pituitary

Fourth ventricle

Medulla oblongata

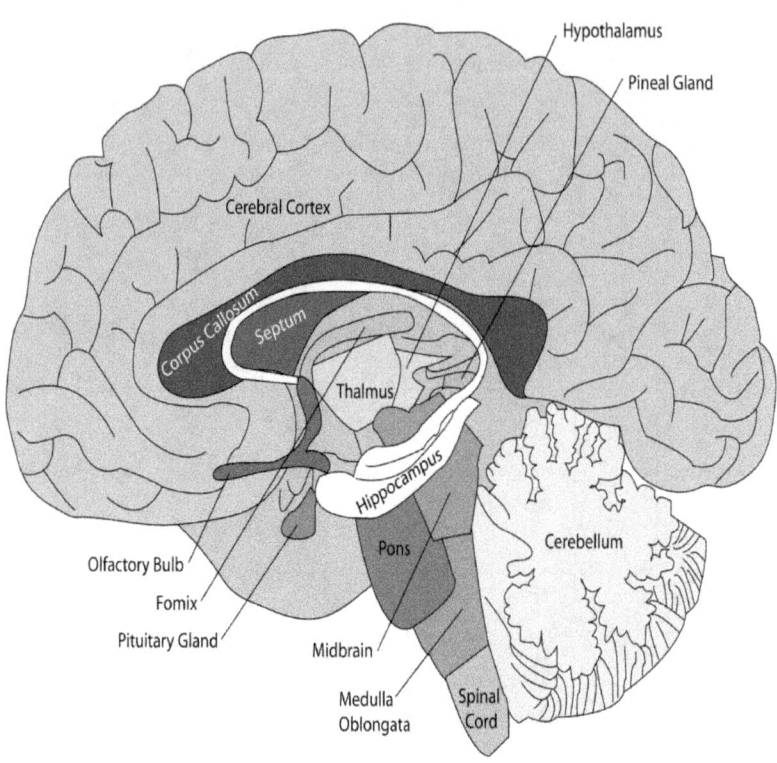

Hypothalamus

Pineal Gland

Cerebral Cortex

Corpus Callosum

Septum

Thalmus

Hippocampus

Olfactory Bulb

Fomix

Pituitary Gland

Midbrain

Medulla Oblongata

Spinal Cord

Pons

Cerebellum

Median section of the brain

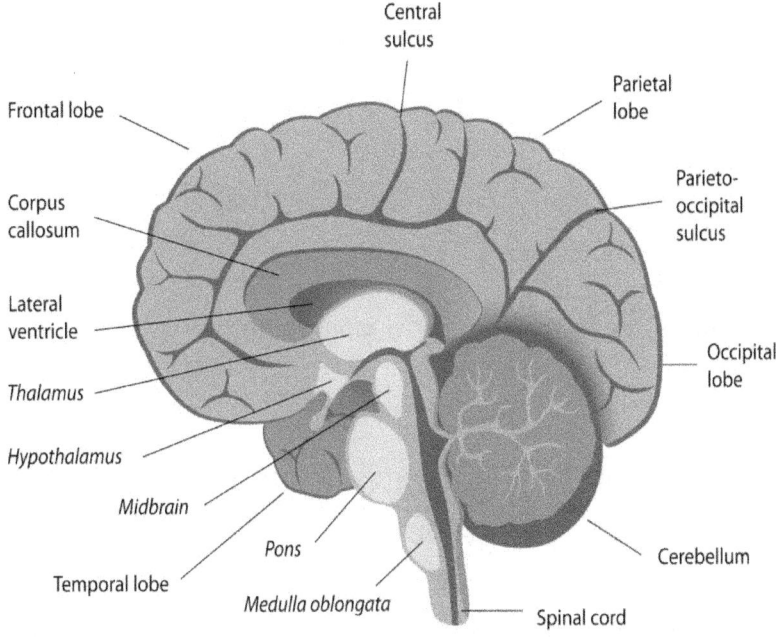

Central
sulcus

Parietal
lobe

Frontal lobe

Parieto-
occipital
sulcus

Corpus
callosum

Lateral
ventricle

Occipital
lobe

Thalamus

Hypothalamus

Midbrain

Pons

Cerebellum

Temporal lobe

Medulla oblongata

Spinal cord

Chapter 10 – Questions

1. Which of the following is not a major region of the brain?
a. cerebrum
b. cerebellum
c. brainstem
d. diencephalon
e. ventricles

2. The bulk of the brain is made of what region?
a. cerebrum
b. cerebellum
c. brainstem
d. diencephalon
e. ventricles

3. What is the name of the depression separating the hemispheres of the cerebrum?
a. central sulcus
b. longitudinal fissure
c. central depression
d. lateral sulcus
e. none of the above

4. Which lobe of the cerebrum is responsible for voluntary motor function?
a. frontal
b. parietal
c. occipital
d. temporal

5. Which lobe of the cerebrum is responsible for sensory perception?
a. frontal
b. parietal
c. occipital
d. temporal

6. Which lobe of the cerebrum is responsible for interpreting vision?
a. frontal
b. parietal
c. occipital
d. temporal

7. Which lobe of the cerebrum is responsible for interpreting hearing?
a. frontal
b. parietal
c. occipital
d. temporal

8. At the bottom of the longitudinal fissure there is a connection between the left and right halves of the brain. This connection is?
a. midbrain
b. thalamus
c. corpus callosum
d. dura mater
e. gyri

9. The part of the brain deep to the occipital bone is?
a. cerebrum
b. cerebellum
c. brainstem
d. diencephalon

e. ventricles

10. The part of the brain responsible for coordinated skeletal muscle activity is?
a. cerebrum
b. cerebellum
c. brainstem
d. diencephalon
e. ventricles

11. Inside of the cerebellum is a mylineated area which looks like a tree. This is the?
a. corpus callosum
b. ventricles
c. folia
d. arbor vitae
e. grey matter

12. The bulk of the diencephalon is made up of the?
a. thalamus
b. hypothalamus
c. epithalamus
d. subthalamus

13. The only sensation which doesn't pass through the thalamus is?
a. taste
b. touch
c. smell
d. pain
e. hearing

14. The most superior part of the brainstem is?
a. pons

b. midbrain

c. medulla oblongata

d. thalamus

e. pia mater

15. Of the three meninges, which is the most superficial?

a. dura mater

b. arachnoid mater

c. pia mater

d. thalamus

e. pons

16. Of the three meninges , which is bound tightly to the surface of the brain?

a. dura mater

b. arachnoid mater

c. pia mater

d. thalamus

e. pons

17. The fluid filled cavities holding cerebrospinal fluid are?

a. corpus callosum

b. ventricles

c. folia

d. arbor vitae

e. grey matter

18. The pineal gland regulates?

a. heart rate

b. ventilation

c. production of cerebrospinal fluid

d. sleep/wake cycles

e. none of the above

19. Visual and auditory reflexes are located within what part of the brain?

a. cerebrum

b. medulla oblongata

c. midbrain

d. corpus callosum

e. diencephalon

20. Which cranial nerve doesn't control a muscle of the eye?

a. optic

b. oculomotor

c. trochlear

d. abducent

21. Which cranial nerve is involved with our sense of smell?

a. olfactory

b. trochlear

c. facial

d. vagus

e. hypoglossal

22. Which cranial nerve is sensory from the face?

a. optic

b. oculomotor

c. trigeminal

d. facial

e. accessory

23. The trapezius muscle is controlled through what nerve?

a. optic

b. oculomotor

c. trigeminal

d. facial

e. accessory

24. The sternocleidomastoid muscle is controlled through what nerve?

a. optic

b. oculomotor

c. trigeminal

d. facial

e. accessory

25. Most facial muscles are controlled through what nerve?

a. optic

b. oculomotor

c. trigeminal

d. facial

e. accessory

26. Our sense of hearing is conducted through what nerve?

a. vestibulocochlear

b. glossopharyngeal

c. vagus

d. abducent

e. trigeminal

27. Our sense of balance (equilibrium) is conducted through what nerve?

a. vestibulocochlear

b. glossopharyngeal

c. vagus

d. abducent

e. trigeminal

28. If an individual was unable to open their eyes, you would suspect damage to what nerve?
a. optic
b. oculomotor
c. trigeminal
d. facial
e. accessory

29. If an individual suddenly lost their ability to focus on objects, you would suspect damage to what nerve?
a. optic
b. oculomotor
c. trigeminal
d. facial
e. accessory

30. If an individual suddenly lost vision, due to cranial nerve damage, you would suspect damage to what nerve?
a. optic
b. oculomotor
c. trigeminal
d. facial
e. accessory

31. What part of the brainstem is connected to the spinal cord?
a. midbrain
b. pons
c. medulla oblongata
d. corpus callosum
e. cerebrum

32. An individual who has lost temperature control within the body has probably damaged the?

a. midbrain

b. pons

c. medulla oblongata

d. hypothalamus

e. epithalamus

33. Pills working to suppress the appetite probably work on what part of the brain?

a. midbrain

b. pons

c. medulla oblongata

d. hypothalamus

e. epithalamus

34. What part of the brain regulates the pituitary gland?

a. midbrain

b. pons

c. medulla oblongata

d. hypothalamus

e. epithalamus

35. The white matter of the cerebrum is composed of?

a. neuron cell bodies

b. dendrites

c. axons and myelin

d. astrocytes

e. ependymal cells

36. The grey matter of the cerebrum is composed of?

a. neuron cell bodies and dendrites

b. cranial nerves

c. axons and myelin

d. astrocytes

e. ependymal cells

37. If someone has a tooth ache, which cranial nerve is responsible for conducting the sensation back to the cerebrum?
a. optic
b. oculomotor
c. trigeminal
d. facial
e. accessory

38. If a person lost their vision, due to cerebral damage, what lobe of the cerebrum was damaged?
a. frontal
b. parietal
c. occipital
d. temporal

39. If a person can no longer rotate their head, what cranial nerve may have been damaged?
a. optic
b. oculomotor
c. trigeminal
d. facial
e. accessory

CHAPTER 10 – Answers to multiple choice questions.

1. E
2. A
3. B
4. A
5. B
6. C
7. D
8. C
9. B
10. B
11. D
12. A
13. C
14. B
15. A
16. C
17. B
18. D
19. C
20. A
21. A
22. C
23. E
24. E
25. D
26. A
27. A
28. B
29. B
30. A

31. C
32. D
33. D
34. D
35. C
36. A
37. C
38. C
39. E

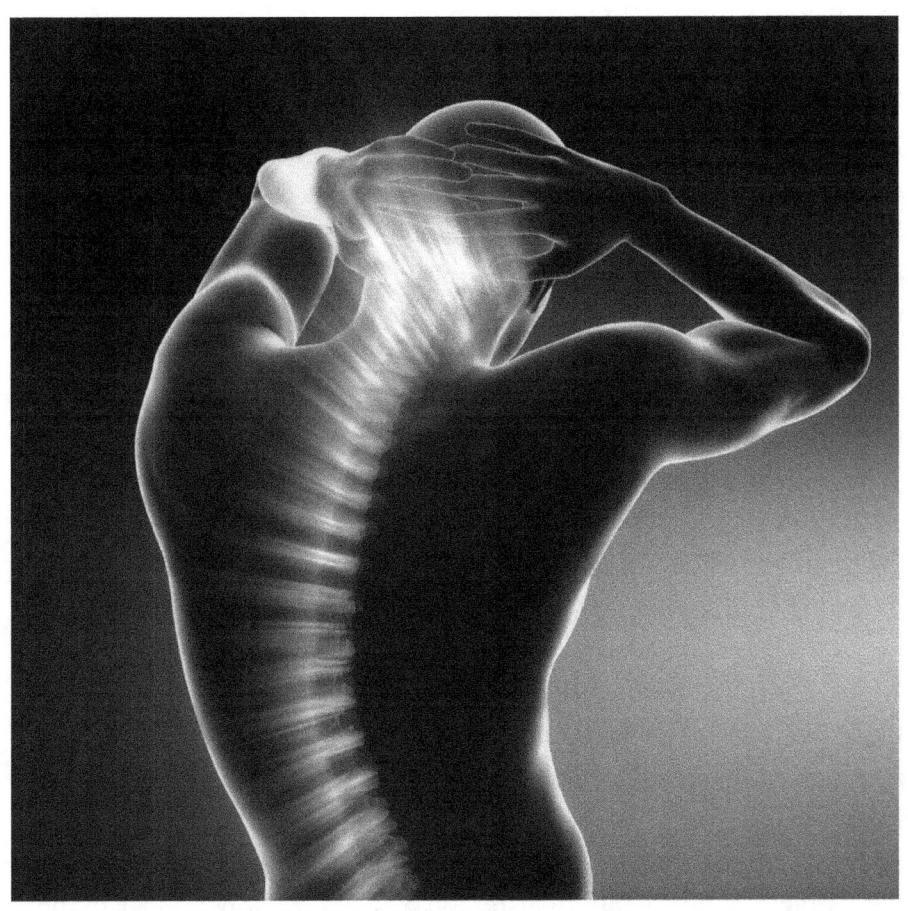

CHAPTER 11 – Spinal Cord

The spinal cord is our connection between the brain and the rest of the body. The spinal cord begins inferior to the medulla oblongata, which is the inferior portion of the brainstem. The spinal cord will extend in an inferior direction through the foramen of the vertebrae. These hard vertebrae protect the spinal cord from injury. The spinal cord will end around the second lumbar vertebrae. The inferior part of the spinal cord is called the conus medullaris. Even though the spinal cord ends at L2 the nerves extending off of it, do not. Many nerves extend in an inferior direction off the conus medullaris and these nerves are collectively called the cauda equina. Cauda means tail in Latin and equine means horse. Someone thought that the nerves look like a horse tail.

As the spinal cord extends in an inferior direction, it gradually gets smaller in diameter. Look at the foramen of the vertebrae and you will see in the cervical region the foramen is large and the foramen of the lumbar vertebrae is small. There are also two thick regions of the spinal cord. The most superior of the two is the cervical enlargement. This thick spot is a region where many axons are coming in and going out to the upper limbs. The inferior enlargement is the lumbar enlargement, where axons from the lower limbs are coming in and out.

Along the spinal cord there are 62 spinal nerves, 31 on each side of the spinal cord. The first spinal nerve exits from the foramen magnum of the occipital bone, many others exit through the intervertebral foramen between the vertebrae and some through the sacral foramen. In the cervical region there are 8 spinal nerves, in the thoracic region 12, lumbar region 5, sacral region 5 and 1 in the coccygeal.

When looking at a cross section of the spinal cord, you can easily see two regions, the white matter and grey matter. White matter is always axons and myelin sheath coverings. The white matter is superficial in the spinal cord, which is the opposite of what you see in the brain. The grey matter is always the nonmylineated areas of dendrites and neuron cell bodies (somas). The spinal cord has a deep depression at the front called the anterior median fissure. By finding this deep depression, you will always know what is the anterior and posterior aspect of the spinal cord.

Much of the area of a spinal cord is white matter. So much of the spinal cord is composed of axons, conducting action potentials up (sensory) and down (motor) the spinal cord. The white matter is separated into three columns, while the grey matter is separated into three horns. The columns and horn are named by their position; anterior, posterior and lateral.

As a spinal nerve approaches the spinal cord, it will split into a dorsal and ventral root. The dorsal root will contain a ganglion (a collection of neuron cell bodies outside of the central nervous system). This ganglion will contain the cell bodies for sensory neurons.

The spinal cord is surrounded by the same three meninges seen around the brain. The dura mater is always the superficial, thickest layer. The arachnoid mater is the meninge in the middle and the pia mater is the deepest layer, bound tightly to the spinal cord.

Our reflexes are located within our spinal cord. A reflex is an automatic (autonomic) response to an outside stimulus. We have reflexes to prevent us from being damaged is some way. Most reflexes have five components to them: 1. Sensory receptor 2. Sensory neuron 3. Interneuron 4. Motor neuron 5. Effector organ. The sensory receptor will detect a stimulus, such as pain. The sensory neuron will conduct the action potential from the sensory receptor back to the central nervous system. The interneuron is located between the sensory and motor neuron and will decide what to do about the stimulus. The motor neuron will conduct an action potential out away from the central nervous system to the effector organ. The effector organ will give a response to the stimulus.

When thinking of a reflex, most people think of the withdrawal reflex. This is the automatic response, which withdraws a body part from a painful stimulus. In each reflex there is a different sensory receptor. Make sure you know which sensory receptor goes with each reflex arc. The withdrawal reflex has a pain receptor at its beginning. The pain receptor will be stimulated by damage to the body. When the pain receptor generates and action potential, the sensory receptor will conduct this action potential back to the spinal cord. When the sensory receptor reaches the spinal cord, it will synapse with the interneuron located within the lateral horn of the grey matter. The interneurons can be one of two types: excitatory or inhibitory. Excitatory neurons will cause muscle contraction, while inhibitory will cause muscle relaxation. With the withdrawal reflex the interneuron is of the excitatory type. It will send an action potential out the motor neuron, out to the muscle and cause the muscle to contract. This will withdraw a body part from a painful stimulus. For example, if you touch a hot stove, your biceps brachii will contract and this will remove your finger from the damage.

Another reflex involves protecting our tendons, called the Golgi tendon reflex. The sensory receptor is located within our tendons and detects intense stretching. If a muscle is applying more tension to a tendon than it can take, the Golgi tendon will send an action potential to the sensory neuron and this will synapse with the interneuron. The interneuron will be of the inhibitory type, because you need to inhibit the muscle (stop it) to prevent damage to the tendon. So, the inhibitory interneuron will send an action potential down the motor neuron to the muscle and stop contraction.

We have another reflex within our spinal cord, which gives us our posture. This is called the stretch reflex. The sensory receptor is the muscle spindle. A muscle spindle is a sensory receptor with detects tiny amounts of stretching and we find these within our posture muscles. If the muscle spindle will detect tiny amounts of stretching in our posture muscles, it will send an action potential up a sensory receptor and synapse with a motor neuron, which will keep tension on the muscle. Notice there isn't any interneuron within this reflex. You have probably seen this reflex tested. If a person sits on a table and hangs their lower limbs over it, this reflex can be tested. A physician can take a small hammer and tap the patellar tendon. This will stretch the quadriceps femoris muscles a very small amount. This small amount of stretching is detected by the muscle spindle and will cause the quadriceps muscles to contract. This is what causes the kicking action of the lower limbs at this time.

These are just some of the more discussed nerves and major functions.

Important spinal nerves

1. Phrenic nerve – innervates the diaphragm muscle, which is needed for ventilation.
2. Thoracic nerves – innervate the pectoralis major and minor, serratus anterior, rectus abdominis, external obliques
3. Axillary nerve – innervate deltoid and teres minor
4. Musculocutaneous nerve – innervate biceps brachii, brachialis
5. Ulnar nerve – flexors of hand. Also known as the funny bone.
6. Median nerve – flexors of hand. Associated with carpal tunnel syndrome.
7. Radial nerve – triceps brachii, brachioradialis and extensors of hand. Associated with crutch paralysis.
8. Femoral nerve – quadriceps femoris, sartorius, pectineus
9. Obturator nerve – adductors of thigh
10. Tibial nerve – gastrocnemius and soleus

11. Gluteal nerve – gluteal muscles

Chapter 11 – Questions

1. The inferior tip of the spinal cord is the?
a. lumbar enlargement
b. conus medullaris
c. cauda equine
d. foramen magnum
e. cervical enlargement

2. The nerves extending off the inferior tip of the spinal cord is the?
a. lumbar enlargement
b. conus medullaris
c. cauda equine
d. foramen magnum
e. cervical enlargement

3. Where the axons of the upper limbs enter and leave the spinal cord, it forms a region called?
a. lumbar enlargement
b. conus medullaris
c. cauda equine
d. foramen magnum
e. cervical enlargement

4. Where the axons of the lower limbs enter and leave the spinal cord, it forms a region called?
a. lumbar enlargement
b. conus medullaris
c. cauda equine
d. foramen magnum
e. cervical enlargement

5. The spinal cord meets the brainstem at the?
a. lumbar enlargement
b. conus medullaris
c. cauda equine
d. foramen magnum
e. cervical enlargement

6. How many spinal nerves do humans have?
a. 31
b. 62
c. 12
d. 33
e. 12

7. How many cervical spinal nerves do we have?
a. 8
b. 12
c. 5
d. 1
e. 31

8. How many thoracic spinal nerves do we have?
a. 8
b. 12
c. 5
d. 1
e. 31

9. How many lumbar spinal nerves do we have?
a. 8
b. 12
c. 5
d. 1

e. 31

10. Where is the grey matter of the spinal cord?
a. superficial
b. deep

11. What will be found in the dorsal root of the spinal nerve?
a. dendrites
b. grey matter
c. cauda equine
d. muscle
e. ganglion

12. Where is the white matter of the spinal cord?
a. superficial
b. deep

13. A reflex always begins with a?
a. sensory receptor
b. sensory neuron
c. interneuron
d. motor neuron
e. effector organ

14. What part of a reflex is located within the lateral horn of the grey matter?
a. sensory receptor
b. sensory neuron
c. interneuron
d. motor neuron
e. effector organ

15. What part of a reflex conducts the action potential towards the central nervous system?
a. sensory receptor
b. sensory neuron
c. interneuron
d. motor neuron
e. effector organ

16. What is the sensory receptor for the withdrawal reflex?
a. baroreceptor
b. pain receptor
c. Golgi organ
d. muscle spindle
e. thermoreceptor

17. What is the sensory receptor for the stretch reflex?
a. baroreceptor
b. pain receptor
c. Golgi organ
d. muscle spindle
e. thermoreceptor

18. Which reflex gives us constant tension in our posture muscles?
a. withdrawal reflex
b. Golgi tendon reflex
c. stretch reflex

19. Which reflex will withdraw a body part from a painful stimulus?
a. withdrawal reflex
b. Golgi tendon reflex
c. stretch reflex

20. Which sensory receptor detects small amounts of stretching (tension)?
a. baroreceptor
b. pain receptor
c. Golgi organ
d. muscle spindle
e. thermoreceptor

21. Which sensory receptor detects intense stretching?
a. baroreceptor
b. pain receptor
c. Golgi organ
d. muscle spindle
e. thermoreceptor

22. Tapping the patellar tendon would test which reflex arc?
a. withdrawal reflex
b. Golgi tendon reflex
c. stretch reflex

23. Which nerve innervates (controls) the diaphragm muscle?
a. thoracic
b. obtorator
c. ulnar
d. axillary
e. phrenic

24. Which nerve innervates (controls) the pectoralis major muscle?
a. thoracic
b. obtorator
c. ulnar
d. axillary
e. phrenic

25. Which nerve innervates (controls) the deltoid muscle?
a. thoracic
b. obtorator
c. ulnar
d. axillary
e. phrenic

26. Which nerve innervates (controls) the biceps brachii muscle?
a. thoracic
b. obtorator
c. mulculocutaneous
d. femoral
e. gluteal

27. Which nerve innervates (controls) the adductors of the thigh?
a. thoracic
b. obtorator
c. ulnar
d. axillary
e. phrenic

28. Which nerve is damaged when we hit our funny bone?
a. thoracic
b. obtorator
c. ulnar
d. axillary
e. phrenic

29. Carpal tunnel syndrome is associated with what nerve?
a. median
b. tibial
c. radial

d. axillary
e. thoracic

CHAPTER 11 – Answers to multiple choice questions.

1. B
2. C
3. E
4. A
5. D
6. B
7. A
8. B
9. C
10. B
11. E
12. A
13. A
14. C
15. B
16. B
17. D
18. C
19. A
20. D
21. C
22. C
23. E
24. A
25. D
26. C
27. B
28. C
29. A

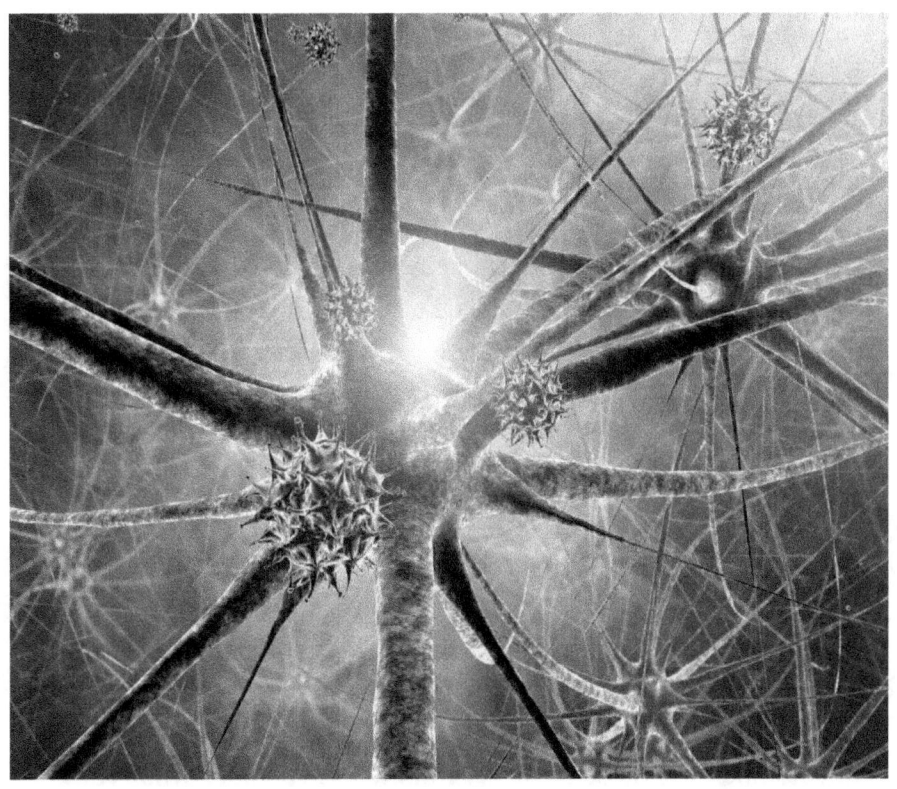

CHAPTER 12 – Sympathetic and Parasympathetic Nervous System

The autonomic nervous system has three subdivisions: sympathetic, parasympathetic and enteric. The sympathetic and parasympathetic are two very important divisions. These two divisions connect too many structures within the body and largely control many of our autonomic functions. The enteric division will be covered with the digestive system.

The sympathetic division is also called the "fight or flight" division. This group of neurons is responsible for all of the changes you see during times of physical activity, stress or strong emotions. Think about what happens to your heart rate, ventilation and blood flow, during physical activity. Our heart beats faster and harder, or ventilation speed increases and more blood flow to the organs needed for physical activity. The sympathetic division causes changes by releasing norepinephrine at the synapses of the tissues. The receptors for norepinephrine are called adrenergic receptors.

The parasympathetic division is also called the "rest and relaxation" division. This group of neurons is responsible for all of the changes you see during times of resting, sleeping or eating. This division of the nervous system will be doing the opposite of what the sympathetic does. The parasympathetic division causes changes by releasing acetylcholine at the synapses of the tissues. The receptors for acetylcholine are called cholinergic receptors.

To understand how these two divisions work, consider what you need for physical activity. The heart, lungs and skeletal muscle are some very important organs. The sympathetic division will enhance the activity of these organs. If you prefer to think of this as speeding them up and causing them to work more, that is essentially correct. Another big change seen during physical activity is a change in blood flow. The sympathetic division will increase the quantity of blood going to the heart, lungs and skeletal muscles being used.

Don't forget that as some organs are being enhanced, other organs are being inhibited. So, don't think of the sympathetic division as only stimulating organs, it inhibits others at the same time. We have a limited amount of blood in our body, so if more blood is being sent to some organs, then less must be sent to others. The sympathetic division will inhibit blood flow to organs not needed for physical activity, like the GI tract. Since we don't need our stomach and intestines for physical activity, the blood flow to them is inhibited by the sympathetic division. For example, sometimes as we run our side starts to hurt. This pain is not in our muscles but in our intestines. When someone starts to run the blood flow to the lower limbs increases. At the same time the blood flow to organs not needed for physical activity decreases. Our side hurts because the intestines are not receiving enough blood to supply them with adequate amounts of oxygen. When an organ is not receiving enough oxygen, it will let you know by hurting. Think about how the heart will hurt when someone is having a heart attack.

Let's consider some organs and the effects of these two divisions.

Organ	Sympathetic	Parasympathetic
Heart	increased heart rate	decreased heart rate
Lungs	faster ventilation	slower ventilation
Stomach	decreased activity	increased activity
Arrector pili	contraction	relaxation
Salivary glands	inhibits salivation	increases salivation

As norepinephrine is released by the sympathetic division, this chemical will bind to specific receptors called adrenergic receptors. Adrenergic receptors come in 4 types: alpha1, alpha2, beta1 and beta2. When you study pharmacology, you will learn the specifics of each receptor type. One of these receptors is commonly mentioned when you hear TV commercials for blood pressure medications. Often beta blockers are mentioned in these commercials. Consider what a beta blocker does, it prevents norepinephrine from working at the receptor sites on the cardiac muscle. Since norepinephrine works to raise blood pressure, a beta blocker would keep the norepinephrine from working, which will help lower blood pressure.

The parasympathetic division releases acetylcholine onto cholinergic receptors. Cholinergic receptors come in 2 types: muscarinic and nicotinic. The muscarinic receptors get their name from a chemical found in some mushrooms. This chemical in the mushrooms will mimic the effects of acetylcholine. What happens when acetylcholine is released onto the heart? The heart will slow its contractions and this will lower blood pressure. If someone were to eat these mushrooms with the acetylcholine like chemical in it, what might happen to them? Their heart might stop is they eat enough of them. This is why you don't eat wild mushrooms.

The other receptor is the nicotinic, obviously getting its name from nicotine. We all know nicotine is found in tobacco and many people are addicted to this chemical. Nicotine will mimic the effects of acetylcholine in many parts of the body, resulting in heart, pulmonary and many other problems.

Chapter 12 – Questions

1. Which division of the nervous system is also called the fight or flight division?
a. sympathetic
b. parasympathetic
c. enteric
d. autonomic
e. central

2. Which division of the nervous system is also called the rest and relaxation division?
a. sympathetic
b. parasympathetic
c. enteric
d. autonomic
e. central

3. The sympathetic division releases what chemical onto target tissues?
a. acetylcholine
b. serotonin
c. norepinephrine
d. all of the above
e. none of the above

4. The sympathetic division of the nervous system would stimulate what organ?
a. stomach
b. kidneys
c. small intestine
d. heart

e. hair growth

5. The sympathetic division would inhibit what?
a. heart
b. muscles of ventilation
c. blood flow to skeletal muscles
d. all of the above
e. none of the above

6. The sympathetic division would do what to salivation?
a. stimulate
b. inhibit
c. nothing

7. The parasympathetic division would do what to heart rate?
a. stimulate
b. inhibit
c. nothing

8. The parasympathetic division would do what to small intestine activity?
a. stimulate
b. inhibit
c. nothing

9. The sympathetic division would do what to the arrector pili muscles in the skin?
a. stimulate
b. inhibit
c. nothing

10. Which is not an adrenergic receptor?
a. alpha1

b. alpha2

c. beta1

d. beta2

e. muscarinic

11. Which is not a cholinergic receptor?

a. muscarinic

b. nicotinic

c. beta1

12. What will the sympathetic division do to blood flow to heart, lungs and skeletal muscles during times of physical activity or stress?

a. stimulate

b. inhibit

c. nothing

13. If a drug is taken which mimics acetylcholine, you would expect the heart rate to do what?

a. increase

b. decrease

c. no effect

CHAPTER 12 – Answers to multiple choice questions.

1. A
2. B
3. C
4. D
5. E
6. B
7. B
8. A
9. A
10. E
11. C
12. A
13. B

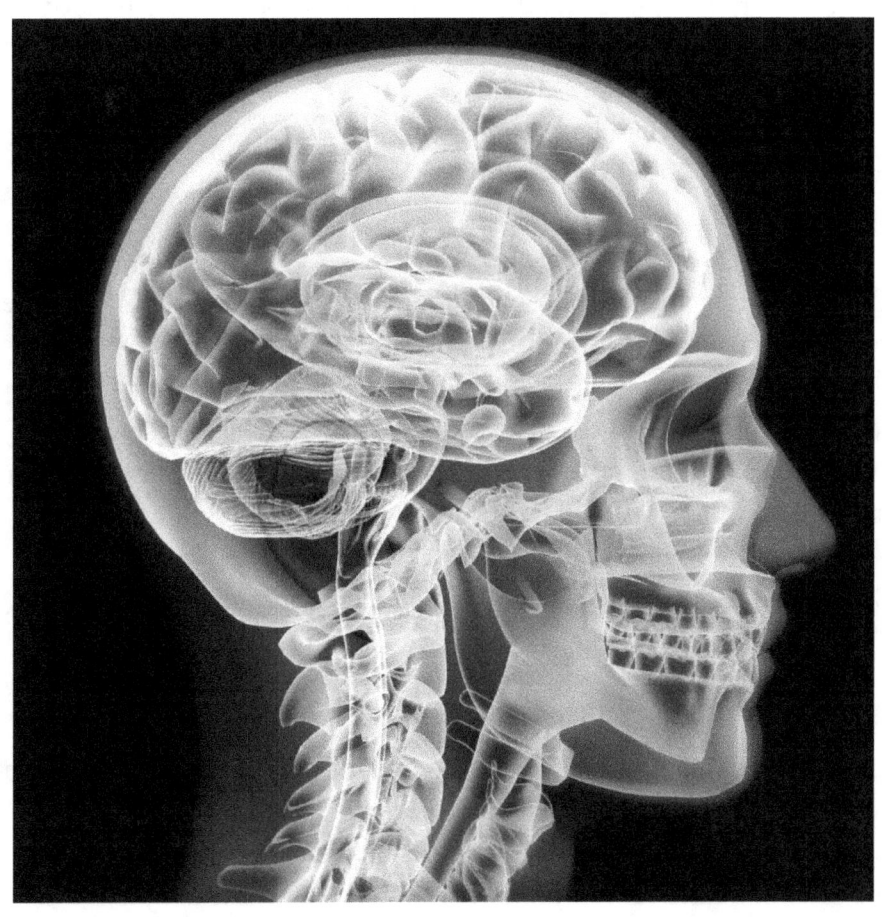

CHAPTER 13 - Senses

A sensation is our brains interpretation of information about our body or environment. We are constantly receiving information about our body and environment and most of this information we aren't consciously aware of. Most of what our brain is doing is happening without our conscious thought. We are constantly receiving signals from within our body and the environment around us. The brain will interpret these action potentials being received from sensory receptors and decide what to do about the. Much of this is to maintain homeostasis, but more is involved.

Sensory receptors can be categorized in many ways. One of the most commonly used ways is to divide them into general senses and special senses.

General senses are senses found in many parts of the body. We have sensory receptors for touch, pain, tickle, itch, etc., in many regions of the body. Special senses are senses we have in one specific region of the body. We only see with our eyes, hear with our ears, smell with our nose, taste with our tongue and have balance with our inner ears. Don't forget the difference between the two.

Senses can also be categorized by the type of stimuli they detect. These are the:
1. Chemoreceptors – These are receptors which detect chemicals. Our sense of smell and taste are examples of chemoreceptors. We are smelling chemicals in the air we inhale and we taste chemicals in what we eat. We have other chemoreceptors within our body. Our hypothalamus has chemoreceptors for blood sugar. Other parts of the brain regulate carbon dioxide and oxygen. These are all chemoreceptors.

2. Photoreceptors – Photoreceptors detect light and give us our ability to see.

3. Thermoreceptors – Thermoreceptors detect changes in temperature, so we know what hot and cold are.

4. Mechanoreceptors – A mechanoreceptor always involves movement, which is what mechanical stimulation is. Our sense of

hearing, balance and many types of touch receptors work in this way.

5. Nociceptors – These are also called pain receptors. If the body is damaged in any way, these receptors will let us know.

6. Osmoreceptors – These are located within the hypothalamus and detect changes in osmolality. Osmolality is the number of particles in solution, basically these are viscosity receptors. If the hypothalamus detects that osmolality is too high, then this means our blood is too thick. When our blood is too thick, we get thirsty. Drinking water will thin our blood back to normal.

7. Baroreceptors – Baroreceptors detect changes in pressure. You can also think of these are stretch receptors, because when pressure increases, structures are stretched. You are consciously aware of the baroreceptors in our stomach and bladder. Others can be found in our arteries, telling our brain what our blood pressure is. The more blood our heart pumps the more this blood stretches our arteries. As the arteries stretch more, they send action potentials to the brain more frequently. This increase in frequency is interpreted as an increase in blood pressure.

8. Proprioreceptors – These are also called tension receptors. These receptors are found in our tendons, detecting muscle tension. If you close your eyes, you can still tell where your hand is. You know when it is down by your side or if it is high above your head, even if you can't see your hand. When your hand is at your side the deltoid muscle isn't applying tension to its attached tendon, but the more you contract the deltoid the more tension it applies to the tendon. This increase in tension allows you to perceive body position.

Adaptation is a functional characteristic exhibited by some sensory receptors. Adaptation refers to the lessening of a sensation over time. Think about if you get close to someone who is wearing perfume. At first the sense of smell is strong and then over time the sensation lessens. Our sense of smell and taste are good examples of senses which exhibit adaptation. Other receptors like pain receptors don't exhibit adaptation. Our body doesn't want a pain receptor to adapt, because if it did, we would forget about things damaging our body.

Other receptors we have detect stimuli from within the body. These receptors are called interorecetors or visceroreceptors. A visceroreceptor is located deep within the body for detection of pain and pressure. Sensory receptors found superficially in the body are exteroreceptors. These receptors are found in the integumentary system and give us information about what is happening around us.

The special senses are smell, taste, vision, hearing and balance (equilibrium).
1. Smell (olfaction) - Our sense of smell takes place in the superior regions of the nasal cavity. Olfactory neurons located within a layer of olfactory epithelium will respond to chemicals being drawn in as we breathe. As we draw air in, we bring chemicals in with the air. These chemicals will stick to the moist mucus environment and diffuse through it. These chemicals will reach the chemoreceptors of smell and generate action potentials. The action potentials will travel back to the brain and our brain will interpret these action potentials as smell.

2. Taste (gustatation) – Our tongue has four different structures located on it called papillae. Papillae are categorized by their shape. The most numerous of the papillae are the filiform. These structures

are the only papillae which don't have taste buds associated with them. The fungiform papillae are the scattered red dots we see on our tongue. The vallate papillae are found on the posterior part of the tongue and the last type is foliate.

Papillae	shape
Filiform	round like a pipe
Fungiform	mushroom shape
Vallate	large and walled
Foliate	leaf shape

Our tastes come in five primary forms: sweet, sour, salty, bitter and umami. The last taste umami refers to the tastes of meats and cheeses. Of these tastes bitter is the strongest and can have an emotional response associated with it. Think of giving a bitter candy to a baby and what response, do they give. Many babies will make a face and shake their head, when given a bitter candy. Many poisonous materials found in plants have a bitter taste. It is believed we are so sensitive to bitter tastes, so we can avoid poisonous plants.

3. Hearing – Our ear has 3 major regions: external, middle and inner.
a. external ear – The external ear contains several structures. Auricle – this is what we think of as the ear, the outer flexible structure. This outer structure contains the helix which is the ridged portion made of cartilage and the inferior lobule portion. This outer ear works like a funnel to collect sound waves and move them towards the external auditory canal. This tunnel extends through the temporal bone and terminates at the tympanic membrane (ear drum). The tympanic membrane is a thin, sensitive structure which will move when the air around it is moved.

b. middle ear – The middle ear contains three bones called auditory ossicles. The three bones of the middle ear are there for sound amplification. Also in this region is the auditory (Eustachian) tube. This passageway connects the middle ear to the pharynx (throat). When we have pressure on the tympanic membrane, we can yawn or swallow to open this passageway. When we do air will move whatever direction is needed to balance the air pressure on the tympanic membrane. This balancing of pressure will allow us to hear properly again.

In the middle ear are two skeletal muscles called the tensor tympani and the stapedius. These two muscles can pull on the bones of the middle ear to protect our inner ear from loud noises. Remember the bones of the middle ear (auditory ossicles) are there to amplify sound. If these muscles pull on the bones, then they can't move easily. This will prevent sound wave amplification and protect the delicate inner ear structures. The autonomic contraction of these muscles is called the attenuation reflex.

c. inner ear – This region begins at the oval window and extends to the cochlear, vestibule and semicircular canals. The cochlea gives us our sense of hearing, while the vestibule and semicircular canals give us our sense of balance.

4. Balance – The vestibule and semicircular canals give us our sense of balance. Our sense of balance takes place inside hollow chambers of the temporal bone. These chambers are filled with fluid and mechanoreceptors called hair cells. Hair cells are modified microvilli. These microvilli are modified to detect movement. When we tilt our head to one side or we accelerate in a vehicle, the fluid around the hair cells will move. This will move the hair cells, tilting them to one side, which will open up ion channels, resulting in depolarizations.

Imagine you are looking at a pond, filled with lake grass growing up from the bottom. If you throw a rock into the water, you generate waves. These waves will move the grass side to side. This is similar to how the mechanoreceptors of the inner ear work.

5. Vision – Before looking at the eyes, make sure you don't forget the accessory structures of the eyes. The accessory structures are structures you don't see with, but they do assist the eyes.

Eyebrows – The eyebrows shade the eyes and help keep perspiration out of the eyes.

Eyelids (palpebrae) – The eyelids are a protective cover over our eyes. We will blink if something approaches our eyes rapidly and this will cover them. We also blink to keep our eyes moist and clean. The eyelashes are the hairs growing off the eyelids. These hairs can also help to protest the eyes. The inner layers of our eyelids are covered with thin mucous membranes called palpebral conjunctiva layers. These are thin layers of epithelial tissue. Inside of our eyelids is a connective tissue layer called the tarsal plate. This plate gives the eyelids shape and structure.

Lacrimal glands (tear glands) – Our lacrimal glands constantly release moisture onto our eyes to keep them moist. If our eyes get dry, they will become red and irritated. After the moisture moves across our eyes, it collects at the medial canthus (corners). From here the moisture passes through tiny holes at the medial corners of the eyelids. These tiny holes are called puncta and can be seen if you pull your top or bottom eyelid down. The moisture will then pass through the lacrimal bone and down into the nasal cavity. Much of the moisture in our nose, comes from our eyes.

We have a few external eye muscles, we use to open and close our eyes. The orbicularis oculi muscles are sphincter muscles we use to close our eyes. The levator palpebral superioris we use to open our eyes.

At the medial corners of each eye is a pink area of tissue called the caruncle. This is where materials collect as they are moved across the eyes.

When we move our eyes we are using six skeletal muscles. Four of these muscles are rectus (straight) muscles. They originate in the rear of the orbit and insert on the sclera (white) of our eyes. Each rectus muscle is named by its position and moves the eye in that same direction. These four muscles are:
1. superior rectus – found above the eye and causes our gaze to go up.
2. inferior rectus – found below the eye and causes our gaze to go down.
3. medial rectus – found at the medial corner and causes our gaze to come inward.
4. lateral rectus – found at the lateral corner and cause our gaze to go out.

In addition to these four rectus muscles, we also have two oblique muscles. These muscles move our gaze in the opposite direction in which they are located. These two muscles are:
5. superior oblique – found above the eye and cause our gaze to go down.
6. inferior oblique – found below the eye and cause our gaze to go up.

So when we look up, we use what two muscles? The superior rectus and the inferior oblique.

When we look down, we use what two muscles? The inferior rectus and the superior oblique.

When we look to the right, we use what muscles? The lateral rectus in the right eye and the medial rectus in the left eye. Make sure you know how these muscles work together.

Looking at the structures of the eye, let's move anterior to posterior.
1. Cornea – the cornea is the clear, avascular structure seen at the front of our eye. This transparent part of the eye allows light to pass in an anterior to posterior direction, penetrating deeper into the eye. Notice also the dome (concave) shape to the cornea. This shape brings light rays together and this is very important for our vision to work properly.

2. Iris – the iris contains melanin and gives us the color of our eyes: brown, blue, green, etc. The iris is made mostly of smooth muscle. This muscle is arranged into two groups: the sphincter group, which makes our pupil smaller and the dilator group which makes our pupil larger.

3. Pupil – the pupil is not a structure, but a hole in the front of our eyes. The iris around the pupil changes the size of the pupil to regulate how much light enters our eyes. If we have a bright light in our face, we can't see. If we are in a dark room, we can't see. We need just the right amount of light entering our pupil to see properly.

4. Lens – deep to the pupil is the lens, an elastic structure that allows us to focus on objects near or far. We can change the thickness of the lens by using the ciliary body (smooth muscle) located around it. The ciliary body connects to the lens by suspensory ligaments. This smooth muscle will allow the lens to thicken to focus on near objects.

5. Vitreous humor – most of the eye is filled with a fluid called vitreous humor. This humor is a thick fluid, which maintains the proper pressure inside of the eye. The fluid inside of the eye can't be too high or too low or the eye won't focus properly. The fluids of the eye exit the eye through two tiny holes at the anterior, superior regions. These holes are the scleral venous sinuses.

6. Retina – the first structure seen in the posterior region of the eye is the retina. The retina is the photoreceptive layer containing the rods and cones. The rods and cones are the photoreceptive neurons responsible for our vision. The rods work well in dim light conditions, but only give us black and white vision. If we only had rods in our eyes, we wouldn't see color, only shades of grey. The cones give us sharp, color vision, but need more light to work. Each photoreceptive neuron has its own advantage and disadvantage. In the center of the retina, there is a concentration of cones. This region is the fovea centralis and it's where we have our best vision. Vitamin A is needed for retinal production for rods to function properly.

7. Choroid – superficial to the retina is the choroid layer. The choroid layer is very vascular and is responsible for the red eye of a camera flash. When you look into someone's eye with an ophthalmoscope, the blood vessels can be seen in the choroid. All of these blood vessels and axons enter and leave the eye at a region called the optic disc.

8. Sclera – superficial to the choroid is the sclera. The sclera is what is also called the "white of the eye." This is a tough, thick collagenous layer which surrounds and protects the eye. The extrinsic muscles which move the eye have their insertion in the sclera.

Eye Disorders

1. Glaucoma – an increase in intraocular pressure, causing a lack of blood flow through the retina.

2. Hyperopia – when an image focuses behind the retina causing a farsighted condition.

3. Myopia – when an image focuses in front of the retina causing a nearsighted condition.

4. Presbyopia – a loss in flexibility in the lens.

5. Cataracts – a clouding of the lens.

6. Astigmatism – irregularly curved cornea or lens.

7. Diabetic retinopathy – a loss in blood supply due to complications from diabetes.

8. Retinal detachment – when the retina separates from the posterior region of the eye.

Human Eye Anatomy

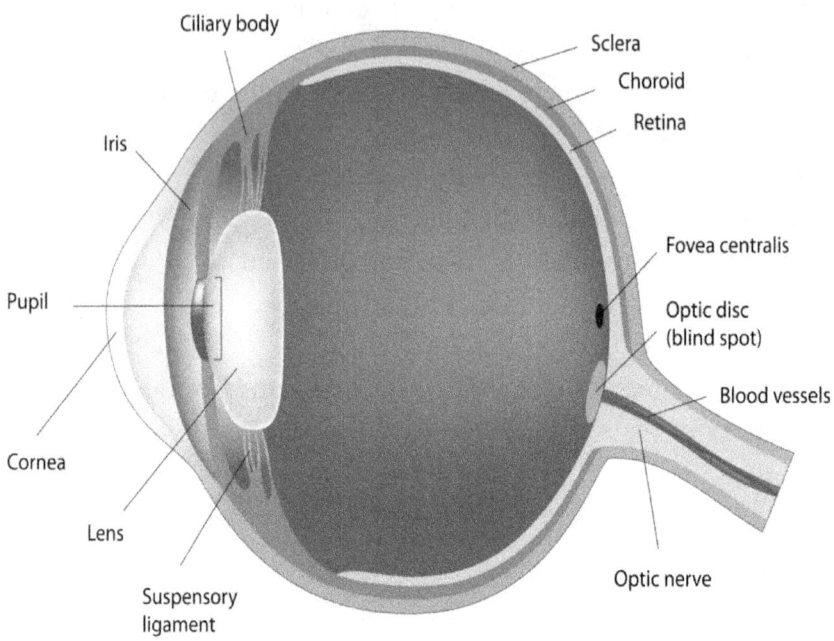

Ciliary body

Sclera

Choroid

Retina

Iris

Fovea centralis

Pupil

Optic disc
(blind spot)

Blood vessels

Cornea

Lens

Suspensory
ligament

Optic nerve

Anatomy of the Ear

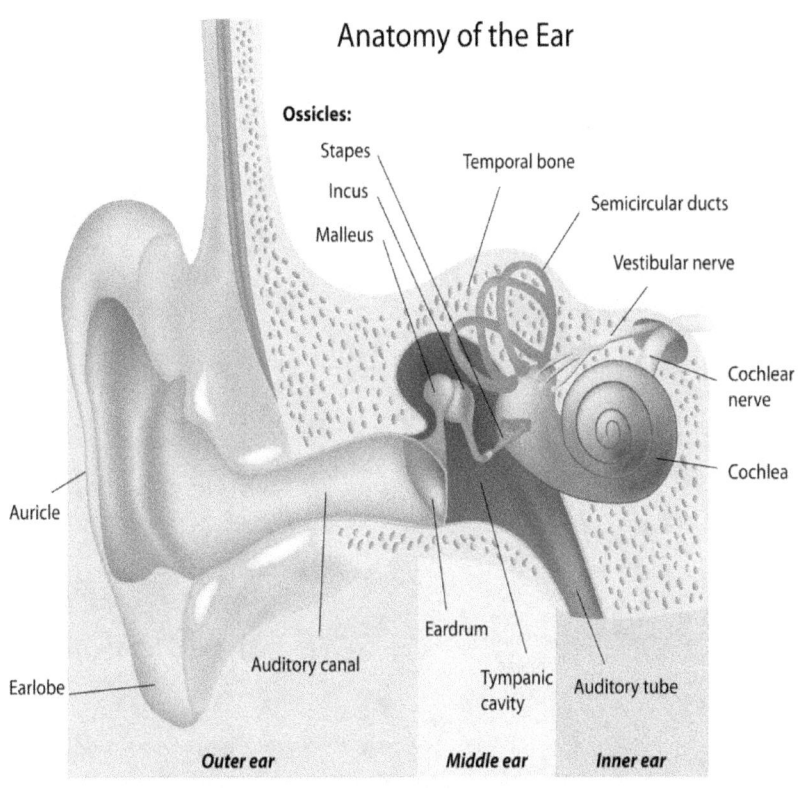

Ossicles:
Stapes
Incus
Malleus

Temporal bone
Semicircular ducts
Vestibular nerve
Cochlear nerve
Cochlea

Auricle
Earlobe
Auditory canal
Eardrum
Tympanic cavity
Auditory tube

Outer ear   *Middle ear*   *Inner ear*

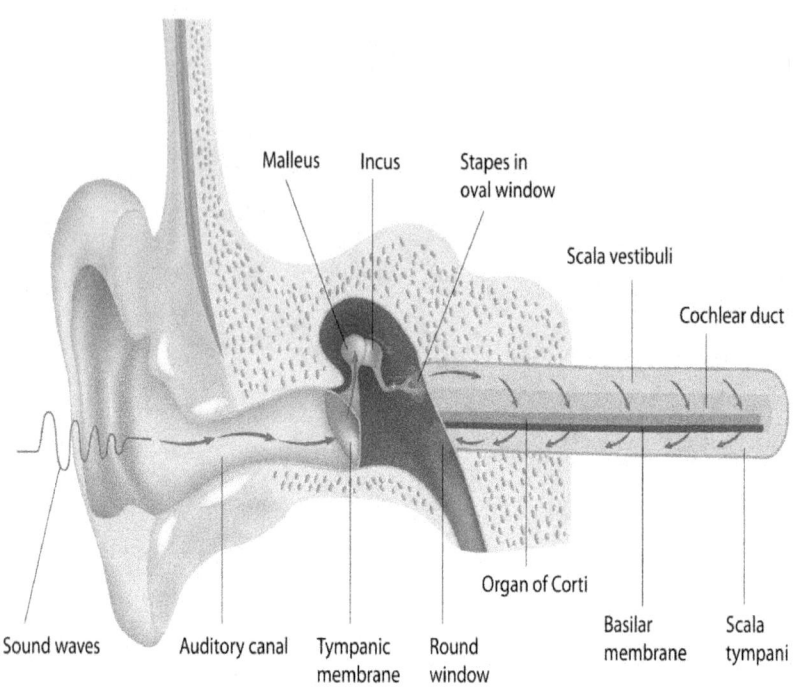

Malleus   Incus   Stapes in oval window

Scala vestibuli

Cochlear duct

Organ of Corti

Sound waves   Auditory canal   Tympanic membrane   Round window   Basilar membrane   Scala tympani

Chapter - 13 Questions

1. What is a general sense?
a. a sense found in one small region of the body
b. a sense found inside the abdominal cavity
c. a sense found over many areas of the body
d. a sense found in the integumentary system
e. all of the above

2. What is a special sense?
a. a sense found in one small region of the body
b. a sense found inside the abdominal cavity
c. a sense found over many areas of the body
d. a sense found in the integumentary system
e. all of the above

3. Our sense of smell and taste are examples of what type of sensory receptor?
a. thermoreceptor
b. mechanoreceptor
c. osmoreceptor
d. chemoreceptor
e. baroreceptor

4. Our sense of touch is an example of what type of sensory receptor?
a. thermoreceptor
b. mechanoreceptor
c. osmoreceptor
d. chemoreceptor

e. baroreceptor

5. Our thirst sensation is detected by what type of sensory receptor?
a. thermoreceptor
b. mechanoreceptor
c. osmoreceptor
d. chemoreceptor
e. baroreceptor

6. Our sense of hearing and balance are what type of sensory receptor?
a. thermoreceptor
b. mechanoreceptor
c. osmoreceptor
d. chemoreceptor
e. baroreceptor

7. Our brain knows our blood pressure through the use of what type of sensory receptor?
a. thermoreceptor
b. mechanoreceptor
c. osmoreceptor
d. chemoreceptor
e. baroreceptor

8. We can detect hot and cold temperatures through the use of what type of sensory receptor?
a. thermoreceptor
b. mechanoreceptor
c. osmoreceptor
d. chemoreceptor
e. baroreceptor

9. A pain receptor is also called a?
a. osmoreceptor
b. baroreceptor
c. nociceptor
d. proprioreceptor
e. exteroreceptor

10. We can know our body position even if our eyes are closed through the use of what type of sensory receptor?
a. osmoreceptor
b. baroreceptor
c. nociceptor
d. proprioreceptor
e. exteroreceptor

11. The perception of some sensory receptors decreases over time. This is called?
a. resolution
b. adaptation
c. gustatation
d. olfaction
e. summation

12. Which of our papillae is long and cylindrical like a straw?
a. filiform
b. fungiform
c. vallate
d. foliate

13. Which of our papillae is shaped like a mushroom?
a. filiform
b. fungiform
c. vallate

d. foliate

14. Which of our papillae doesn't have taste buds associated with them?
a. filiform
b. fungiform
c. vallate
d. foliate

15. Which of our papillae look like little red dots on our tongue?
a. filiform
b. fungiform
c. vallate
d. foliate

16. Of our 5 primary tastes, which is the strongest?
a. sweet
b. sour
c. salty
d. bitter
e. umami

17. The tympanic membrane is found in the?
a. external ear
b. middle ear
c. inner ear

18. The external auditory canal passes through what bone?
a. frontal
b. sphenoid
c. parietal
d. temporal
e. occipital

19. The external fleshy part of our ear is called the?
a. tympanic membrane
b. auricle
c. round window
d. malleus
e. cochlea

20. The ridged parts of our ear are called?
a. lobule
b. helix
c. semicircular canals
d. vestibule
e. incus

21. We can equalize pressure on the tympanic membrane by moving air through what?
a. external auditory canal
b. semicircular canals
c. cochlea
d. auditory tube
e. all of the above

22. The ear drum is also called the?
a. tympanic membrane
b. auricle
c. round window
d. malleus
e. cochlea

23. The three bones of the middle ear are used for?
a. protection
b. equilibrium

c. balance

d. to balance air pressure

e. sound amplification

24. The Eustachian tube connects the middle ear to the?

a. inner ear

b. outer ear

c. nasal cavity

d. pharynx

e. all of the above

25. The cochlea is responsible for?

a. hearing

b. balance

c. equilibrium

d. air pressure

e. sound amplification

26. The semicircular canals are responsible for?

a. hearing

b. balance

c. air pressure

d. air pressure

e. sound amplification

27. The attenuation reflex performs what function?

a. sound amplification

b. equilibrium

c. prevents sound amplification

d. moves the tympanic membrane

e. balances air pressure

28. The structure between the stapes and the vestibule is the?

a. tympanic membrane
b. round window
c. oval window
d. semicircular canals
e. cochlea

29. The palpebrae are also called the?
a. eyelids
b. eyebrows
c. eyelashes
d. tear glands
e. none of the above

30. The tear glands are also known as the?
a. sebaceous glands
b. ceruminous glands
c. lacrimal glands
d. sweat glands
e. mammary glands

31. Which muscle will turn our gaze up?
a. superior rectus
b. inferior rectus
c. lateral rectus
d. superior oblique
e. medial rectus

32. Which muscle will turn our gaze down?
a. superior rectus
b. inferior rectus
c. lateral rectus
d. inferior oblique
e. medial rectus

33. The superior oblique muscle works together with which muscle?
a. superior rectus
b. inferior rectus
c. lateral rectus
d. medial rectus
e. inferior oblique

34. The inferior oblique muscle works together with which muscle?
a. superior rectus
b. inferior rectus
c. lateral rectus
d. medial rectus
e. inferior oblique

35. Which structure is the most anterior?
a. retina
b. sclera
c. cornea
d. lens
e. iris

36. Which structure contains the rods and cones?
a. retina
b. sclera
c. cornea
d. lens
e. iris

37. Which flexible structure is responsible for focusing on near objects?
a. retina
b. sclera

c. cornea

d. lens

e. iris

38. The dark hole in the front of the eye is the?

a. retina

b. pupil

c. sclera

d. choroid

e. iris

39. What part of the eye controls the size of the pupil?

a. retina

b. pupil

c. sclera

d. choroid

e. iris

40. The muscles which move the eye insert on the?

a. retina

b. pupil

c. sclera

d. choroid

e. iris

41. The vascular layer of the eye is?

a. retina

b. pupil

c. sclera

d. choroid

e. iris

42. The part of our eye which has colored melanin is?

a. retina

b. pupil

c. sclera

d. choroid

e. iris

43. An increase in pressure inside of the eye is commonly known as?

a. glaucoma

b. hyperopia

c. cataracts

d. astigmatism

e. myopia

44. If a person is farsighted they have?

a. glaucoma

b. hyperopia

c. cataracts

d. astigmatism

e. myopia

45. If a person is nearsighted they have?

a. myopia

b. hyperopia

c. presbyopia

d. astigmatism

e. glaucoma

46. A clouding of the lens is?

a. retinal detachment

b. astigmatism

c. myopia

d. glaucoma

e. cataracts

47. An irregularity in the shape of the cornea or lens is?
a. retinal detachment
b. astigmatism
c. myopia
d. glaucoma
e. cataracts

CHAPTER 13 – Answers to multiple choice questions.

1. C
2. A
3. D
4. B
5. C
6. B
7. E
8. A
9. C
10. D
11. B
12. A
13. B
14. A
15. B
16. D
17. A
18. D
19. B
20. B
21. D
22. A
23. E
24. D
25. A
26. B
27. C
28. C
29. A
30. C

31. A
32. B
33. B
34. A
35. C
36. A
37. D
38. B
39. E
40. C
41. D
42. E
43. A
44. B
45. A
46. E
47. B

APPENDIX

Most all texts for Human Anatomy and Physiology have the exact same material in them. The better ones have thousands of illustrations and examples. You can choose the one you prefer or the one your instructor has selected. Below is a list of texts used as a reference.

Marieb, Elaine and Katja Hoehn. Human Anatomy and Physiology. Benjamin-Cummings Pub Co; (May 30, 2006).

Martini, Frederic; William C. Ober, Claire W. Garrison, Kathleen Welch and Ralph T. Hutchings. Fundamentals of Anatomy and Physiology. 5th ed. Prentice Hall College Division. January, 2001.

McKinley, Michael; Valerie O'Loughlin and Theresa Bidle. Anatomy and Physiology. 1ed McGraw Hill Science. January 6, 2012

Patton, Kevin T. and Gary A. Thibodeau. Anatomy & Physiology. 7th ed. Mosby. (February 26, 2009).

Saladin, Kenneth S. Anatomy and Physiology. McGraw Hill Higher Education; 5th edition (February 15, 2009)

Seeley, Rod R., Trent D. Stephens, and Philip Tate. Anatomy & Physiology. 9th ed. Boston, Mass. McGraw-Hill, 2010.

Shier, David; Ricki Lewis and Jackie Butler. Holes Human Anatomy and Physiology. 9th ed. McGraw-Hill. 2009.

Tortora, Gerard J. and Bryan Derrickson. Introduction to the Human Body. 9th ed. John Wiley and Sons, Inc. 2012.

www.ingramcontent.com/pod-product-compliance
Lightning Source LLC
Chambersburg PA
CBHW051446170526
45166CB00001B/137